INTERMITTENT
FASTING
BASICS

INCLUDES 50+ RECIPES

Your Guide to the Essentials of Intermittent Fasting—and How It Can Work for You!

FASTING GUIDELINES

STARTER RECIPES

LIFESTYLE ADJUSTMENTS

LINDSAY BOYERS, CHNC

Adams Media
New York London Toronto Sydney New Delhi

▲adamsmedia

Adams Media
An Imprint of Simon & Schuster, Inc.
57 Littlefield Street
Avon, Massachusetts 02322

Copyright © 2019 by Simon & Schuster, Inc.

All rights reserved, including the right to reproduce this book or portions thereof in any form whatsoever. For information address Adams Media Subsidiary Rights Department, 1230 Avenue of the Americas, New York, NY 10020.

First Adams Media trade paperback edition May 2019

ADAMS MEDIA and colophon are trademarks of Simon & Schuster.

For information about special discounts for bulk purchases, please contact Simon & Schuster Special Sales at 1-866-506-1949 or business@simonandschuster.com.

The Simon & Schuster Speakers Bureau can bring authors to your live event. For more information or to book an event contact the Simon & Schuster Speakers Bureau at 1-866-248-3049 or visit our website at www.simonspeakers.com.

Interior images © Getty Images

Manufactured in the United States of America

10 9 8 7 6 5 4 3 2 1

Library of Congress Cataloging-in-Publication Data has been applied for.

ISBN 978-1-5072-1055-0
ISBN 978-1-5072-1056-7 (ebook)

Many of the designations used by manufacturers and sellers to distinguish their products are claimed as trademarks. Where those designations appear in this book and Simon & Schuster, Inc., was aware of a trademark claim, the designations have been printed with initial capital letters.

The information in this book should not be used for diagnosing or treating any health problem. Not all diet and exercise plans suit everyone. You should always consult a trained medical professional before starting a diet, taking any form of medication, or embarking on any fitness or weight-training program. The author and publisher disclaim any liability arising directly or indirectly from the use of this book.

Always follow safety and commonsense cooking protocols while using kitchen utensils, operating ovens and stoves, and handling uncooked food. If children are assisting in the preparation of any recipe, they should always be supervised by an adult.

Contains material adapted from the following title published by Adams Media, an Imprint of Simon & Schuster, Inc.: *The Everything® Guide to Intermittent Fasting* by Lindsay Boyers, CHNC, copyright © 2018, ISBN 978-1-5072-0841-0.

Contents

Introduction

You may have heard about the health benefits of fasting. Not only does it help you lose weight; it also makes your mind clearer and gives you more energy. But where do you begin?

With the basics.

Intermittent Fasting Basics teaches you everything you need to know about fasting in a quick, easy-to-understand way. Wondering how to set up your fasts? You'll find out how to systematically plan your eating habits. Not sure how to derive the greatest benefit from this practice? You'll see a clear set of guidelines, including various fasting plans so you can select the one that best fits your schedule and your needs. Unsure how to construct a diet that best works with intermittent fasting? This book gives detailed advice about what to eat and drink. Plus, there are more than fifty delicious recipes that will supplement your fasting in a healthy way!

You'll learn the ins and outs of fasting. How you apply this information is up to you. Maybe you want to set a regular schedule of fasting, or maybe you want to fast spontaneously, when the moment moves you. Maybe you want to lose weight as well as address health issues.

No matter what your reasons for intermittent fasting are, this book is here to help you confidently ease into this new lifestyle and apply it to your life—easily and effectively.

1

Getting Started with Intermittent Fasting

As the name implies, intermittent fasting is a lifestyle in which you periodically go without food. This doesn't mean you starve—far from it. Instead, you mix fasting with a healthy diet, being mindful about what you eat and drink in order to promote better health and mental clarity. When you approach it in the right way, intermittent fasting can help you combat diabetes and other conditions related to high blood sugar, as well as everything from insomnia to heart disease. If you're interested in intermittent fasting, the following information can help you get started.

What Is Intermittent Fasting?

Although it may seem like you're hearing a lot more about it recently, intermittent fasting is not a new concept. In fact, fasts have been an important part of history and religion for centuries. Many people are starting to catch on to the health benefits of fasting, from a boost in energy to weight loss and increased mental clarity. Intermittent fasting isn't a specific diet plan. It's a general term that describes an eating pattern in which you alternate between eating and fasting (purposefully going without food for a set period of time). To fully understand intermittent fasting, it's helpful to know the difference between a fed state and a fasted state—the two phases of the digestive system.

The Fed State

A fed, or absorptive, state happens right after a meal or a snack, when your body is digesting the food and absorbing its nutrients. Digestion continues until the broken-down components of your food are transported into your blood, where they travel to the liver, fatty (adipose) tissue, and muscles.

The broken-down components of food first entering your blood causes your blood glucose levels to rise, which then stimulates the beta cells (the specialized cells in your pancreas that produce, store, and release insulin) to release insulin into the blood. The released insulin then attaches to the glucose in your blood and carries it to the cells, where it's used for energy, or carries it to the liver and muscles, where it's converted to glycogen and stored for later use.

The Fasted State

Once the fed state ends, your body enters the fasted, or post-absorptive, state. When you're in the fasted state, approximately four hours after you eat, your body relies on stored glycogen for energy. Glucose levels in the blood drop as the cells begin to use the sugar, and in response to this decrease in glucose, insulin levels drop as well. Because your body likes to maintain blood glucose levels between 70 and 99 milligrams per deciliter, this drop in glucose in the blood triggers the alpha cells of the pancreas to release a hormone called *glucagon*. Glucagon travels to the liver, where it breaks glycogen down into glucose. Once glucose is formed, it's released by the liver and travels to your brain and tissues.

Why Do People Fast?

When it comes to the history of civilization, easy, regular access to food is actually a fairly new concept. Before the Industrial Revolution, people had to rely solely on the land to get food. They couldn't simply take a ride to their nearest grocery store any time they needed to fill their stomachs. Ancient civilizations hunted and gathered as much as they could (and some civilizations around the world today still hunt and gather). But food wasn't always a guarantee. Sometimes the hunters and gatherers would come back with a fresh kill and a load of fresh fruit and berries; other days, especially in times of scarcity, like the winter months, they would come back empty-handed. Although they weren't doing it intentionally, they were essentially fasting on these days. Depending on the time of the year and the skill of the hunters and gatherers, these fasts could last days, weeks, or even months.

Fasting Long Ago

Some ancient civilizations caught on to the benefits of fasting well before modern research. The ancient Greeks believed that fasting could improve cognitive abilities and concentration. And according to Benjamin Franklin, one of America's founding fathers and the claimed inventor of the lightning rod and bifocal glasses, "the best of all medicines are resting and fasting."

Spiritual Fasting

Fasting has also been—and remains—an important part of various religions and spiritual practices around the world. When used for religious purposes, fasting is often described as a cleansing or purification process, but the basic concept is still the same: abstain from eating for a set period of time.

Unlike medical fasting, which is used as a treatment for illness, spiritual fasting is seen as an important catalyst to whole-body wellness, and a wide variety of religions share the belief that fasting has the power to heal. In Buddhism, fasting is a way to practice restraint from acting on human desires, a restraint that Buddhist monks believe is a piece of the puzzle to achieving nirvana. Many Buddhists fast daily, eating food in the morning but abstaining for the rest of the day, until it is time to eat the next morning. In addition to this, Buddhists often embark on a water-only fast for days or weeks.

Maha-shivaratri

In Hinduism, it's believed that denying the physical needs of the body by fasting helps increase spirituality. Although fasting is a regular part of the Hindu religion and is done often, one of the most popular observed fasts is during Maha-shivaratri, or the "Great Night of Shiva." During Maha-shivaratri, devotees fast; take part in ritual baths; visit a temple where they pray; and practice the virtues of honesty, forgiveness, and self-discipline.

In Judaism, there are several reasons to fast, including asking for God's mercy, marking important life events, showing gratitude to God, or mourning; however, if you are doing an individual fast, it is custom to keep the fast private.

Lent

In Christianity, fasting is a way to cleanse the soul so that the body is pure and so that a connection with God can be made. One of the most popular times that Christians fast is Lent, the forty-day period between Ash Wednesday and Easter. In earlier days, those observing Lent gave up food or drink; in more modern times, Christians might still abstain from food or drink but often choose instead to go without a specific thing. This practice is meant to be an acknowledgment of the forty days that Jesus Christ spent in the desert, forced to fast.

Ramadan

Perhaps the most well-known religious fast, Ramadan is a major part of the Muslim religion and the ninth month of the Islamic calendar. During Ramadan, Muslims not only abstain from food and drink from dusk to dawn; they also avoid smoking, sexual relations, and any other activities that may be viewed as sinful. The period of fasting—and the mild dehydration that occurs from lack of fluids—is believed to cleanse the soul of harmful impurities so that the heart can be redirected to spirituality and away from earthly desires. Ramadan is regarded as one of the Five Pillars of Islam.

Medical Fasting

Hippocrates, who's been nicknamed "the father of medicine," introduced fasting as a medical therapy for some of his sick patients as far back as the fifth century B.C.E. One of Hippocrates's famous quotes states that "to eat when you are sick is to feed your sickness." He believed that fasting allowed the body to focus on healing itself, and that forcing food in a diseased state could actually be detrimental to a person's health, because instead of giving the necessary energy to healing, your body would use all of its available energy on digestion. On the other hand, if sick patients abstained from food, digestive processes would shut down and the body would prioritize natural healing.

Fasting As Therapy

Some medical fasts allowed only water and calorie-free tea for up to one month, while others allowed patients to consume 200–500 calories per day. These calories typically came from bread, broths, juices, and milk. The specific details of the fast depended on the person's condition. However, it wasn't until the 1900s that fasting started appearing in scientific journals as an effective medical therapy for obesity and other illnesses; even then, the benefits didn't fully catch on until more recently.

The Science of Fasting

Like any nutritional concept that quickly takes over health and diet communities, intermittent fasting has been accused of being a fad, but the science behind the benefits of fasting is already clear—and growing. There are several theories as to why intermittent fasting works so well, but the most frequently studied—and most proven—benefit has to do with stress.

The word *stress* has been vilified time and time again, but some stress is actually beneficial to your body. For example, exercise is technically a stress to the body (to the muscles and the cardiovascular system, specifically), but this particular stress ultimately makes the body stronger as long as you incorporate the right amount of recovery time into your exercise routine.

According to Dr. Mark Mattson—the senior investigator and lab chief at the Laboratory of Neurosciences at the National Institute on Aging, and a neuroscience professor at Johns Hopkins University School of Medicine—intermittent fasting stresses the body in the same way exercise does. When you deny the body food for a set period of time, it puts the cells under mild stress. Over time, cells adapt to this stress by learning how to cope with it better. When your body is better at dealing with stress, it has an increased ability to resist disease.

How Stress Works

While some types of stress are good for the body, helping it to adapt and grow, other types of stress aren't. It's important to distinguish between good and bad stresses so that you can get a handle on the bad ones. When you're exposed to stress, a part of your brain called the *amygdala* recognizes that stress as a threat to your health. In response to this threat, the amygdala sends a message to another part of your brain, the *hypothalamus*, to release corticotropin-releasing hormone, or CRH. CRH then stimulates yet another part of your brain, the *pituitary gland*, to release adrenocorticotropic hormone, or ACTH. The release of ACTH signals the adrenal glands to produce and release cortisol. The adrenal glands also release adrenaline, which elevates your blood pressure and increases your heart rate. The presence of cortisol helps maintain proper blood pressure and fluid balance while temporarily shutting down some body functions, like digestion, to preserve energy. In this case, once the immediate threat goes away, cortisol levels drop back down and normal body functions are resumed.

Eustress: Short-Lived Stress

Good stress, also referred to as *eustress*, is a mild stress that most people experience on a regular basis. Instead of being harmful to the body, eustress inspires you and propels you to reach a goal or a desired outcome, and it's generally associated with some type of happiness or excitement when that goal is achieved. Examples of eustress include training for an athletic event, working toward a deadline, or practicing for an upcoming performance. Research shows that eustress can actually improve your brain function. The defining characteristic of eustress is that it is short-lasting. Once the goal is met or the project is finished, eustress goes away and your cortisol levels drop back down and normalize, giving your body time to recover.

Distress: Bad Stress

Bad stress, or what is otherwise known as *distress*, is chronic, unrelenting stress that hinders your productivity or gets in the way of your daily life. Instead of pushing you to achieve your goals, distress makes it harder to achieve them. Distress keeps your cortisol and adrenaline levels high, which can lead to weakened adrenal glands and problems with normal hormonal signaling. Some chronic health problems linked to distress include depression, heart disease, weight gain, and a greater susceptibility to illnesses like colds and flus. Examples of distress include toxic romantic relationships, constant work stress, and trauma or death in the family.

However, because everyone reacts differently to certain things and has a different perspective on life, the line between good and bad stress can become blurred. The best way to determine whether something is eustress or distress for you is to ask yourself a few questions: Does it make you feel challenged, yet motivated? If so, it's likely good stress. Does it make you feel overwhelmed, withdrawn, and tired? If so, it's probably bad stress.

Should You Fast?

Fasting is appropriate for most healthy people, but there are certain groups of people who shouldn't fast or who should speak to their healthcare team before starting a fast.

You should not fast if you:

- Are pregnant or breastfeeding
- Are severely underweight or malnourished
- Are under eighteen years of age

You should speak to your healthcare provider before fasting if you:

- Are taking any medications
- Have a history of disordered eating
- Have cortisol dysregulation or are under severe stress
- Have diabetes (type 1 or type 2)
- Have GERD (gastroesophageal reflux disease)
- Have gout

Listen to Your Body

Listen carefully to your body to determine if fasting is right for you. If you're feeling low in energy or light-headed upon standing, you may have to adjust your fasting window or check in with your doctor to make sure your body can regulate your blood sugar properly. Keep in mind that it can take a long time for your body to adjust to your new lifestyle. There is typically a three- to six-week transition period during which your body and your brain adapt to fasting. During this time, you may experience hunger, irritability, weakness, and even loss of libido. This is a normal response, but if symptoms are severe, work with your healthcare provider during these initial stages. If you feel great after the adjustment period, then it's a good sign that your body likes what you're doing. If you feel dizzy, light-headed, or low on energy after this period, then you should stop fasting and speak with your healthcare provider.

Fasting and Diabetes

Fasting can be a challenge for those with diabetes because the body has a harder time regulating blood glucose and insulin levels than it does in people who don't have diabetes. However, research shows that intermittent fasting may be beneficial in helping to return glucose levels to normal. The biggest concern when it comes to fasting and diabetes is hypoglycemia, or low blood sugar.

Get Your Doctor's Approval

If you have diabetes, make sure that you have your doctor's approval and supervision before starting any type of fast. If your doctor approves intermittent fasting, familiarize yourself with the symptoms of low blood sugar and have a plan in place for treating your blood sugar levels if they get too low. If blood sugar levels exceed 300 milligrams per deciliter or drop below 70 milligrams per deciliter, stop the fast immediately and apply the proper treatment.

Hypoglycemia

Hypoglycemia is more likely to occur in those with type 1 diabetes than those with type 2 diabetes. Signs of hypoglycemia include:

- Anxiety
- Fatigue
- Hunger
- Increased sweating
- Irregular heartbeat
- Irritability
- Pale skin
- Shakiness

Severe hypoglycemia may cause:

- Abnormal behavior or mental confusion
- Blurred vision
- Confusion
- Loss of consciousness
- Seizure

If you experience any of these symptoms, seek medical attention.

Get Control of Chronic Conditions

The stress that fasting puts on the body can be categorized as eustress for most people. It's mild, and it results in health benefits that can push you to keep going to achieve your ultimate goals. However, if you're under chronic distress already, you'll want to get that under control before you incorporate intermittent fasting into your routine. In the case of chronic stress, your body is continuously pumping out cortisol. When cortisol levels stay elevated for an extended period of time, it can lead to:

- Anxiety
- Depression
- Difficulty sleeping
- Digestive issues
- Headaches
- Heart disease
- Problems with memory and concentration
- Weight gain

Over time chronic stress also affects the function of your adrenal glands negatively and makes it harder for them to regulate hormones properly.

If you're already under a great deal of chronic stress, getting your cortisol levels under control and your adrenal glands working properly before beginning to fast is extremely important. You can reduce cortisol levels by meditating; avoiding coffee; getting enough sleep; following a clean, healthy diet for a period of time before incorporating fasting; and avoiding excessive exercise. Low-impact, meditative exercises like yoga can be helpful.

Preparing to Fast

With the exception of spontaneous fasting (which we'll talk about later), most types of intermittent fasting require some preparation. One of the most important things you can do to prepare for your fast is to develop a plan. What type of intermittent fasting will you be doing? During which days and times will you fast? What is your official start date? It's helpful to write out a schedule for yourself and keep it where you can see it all the time. You can even set timers on your phone to go off when it's time to begin your fast and when it's time to start eating again. But you also don't have to jump into a set fasting schedule right away; you can ease yourself in slowly to get the hang of it.

Do Yoga

In a study conducted by the Yoga Research Society and the Sidney Kimmel Medical College at Thomas Jefferson University, researchers found that cortisol levels dropped significantly after a fifty-minute yoga class that included popular yoga poses like the Tree Pose, Plow Pose, and Locust Pose. Researchers believe that this drop in cortisol is due in part to the activation of the relaxation response through the holding of poses and deep breathing. This relaxation response shuts off the stress cascade, and as a result, stress hormones are naturally reduced. High cortisol levels are also common in those with depression. A study published in the *Indian Journal of Psychiatry* found that yoga may help shut off the stress response in the hypothalamus section of the brain, which can bring relief to those with depression. In fact, the study found that yoga dropped cortisol levels better than antidepressants did.

Practice Meditation

Research suggests that daily meditation doesn't just feel good in the moment: it can actually alter the brain's neural pathways, reducing anxiety and making you more resilient and resistant to stress. There's no right or wrong way to meditate, so don't let your preconceived notions about what meditation is supposed to be deter you from starting your own routine. If you're new to meditation, you can start by following along with some guided meditations. You can access thousands of meditation videos online to help get you started.

Two Types of Meditation

Generally speaking, there are two types of meditation:

1. In concentration meditation you focus your consciousness on a single point (for many people this means repeating a short phrase, called a mantra).

2. In mindfulness meditation you allow various thoughts and sensations to drift through your mind, examining each of them without judgment.

Either of these can be useful in preparing your mind for intermittent fasting.

Try Deep Breathing

Meditation and deep breathing go hand in hand, but you can do some quick deep-breathing exercises on your own, too, whenever you feel stress building up—or even when you don't and you want to stay ahead of it. When you're stressed, you tend to take quick, shallow breaths that come from your chest rather than your abdomen. When you breathe deeply from your abdomen instead, you take in more oxygen, which helps you feel less anxious, less short of breath, and more relaxed. Learning how to take deep breaths takes practice, but the following steps will make it easy for you to become a pro deep-breather in no time:

1. Sit up straight or lie on your back somewhere comfortable. Put one hand on your chest and the other on your abdomen.

2. Take a deep breath in through your nose. You should feel the hand on your abdomen rise, but the hand on your chest should move very little.

3. Exhale through your mouth, pushing out as much air as you can.

4. Repeat this process until you feel your body start to relax

Listen to Music

You know that feeling when your favorite song comes on and you start to sing along and immediately feel better? There's science behind that. Research shows that regardless of what mood you're in, listening to music that you love can lower your cortisol levels. Although any music that you love can have a stress-lowering effect, classical music shows great results. Listening to classical music can lower stress hormones, decrease blood pressure, and slow down both your pulse and your heart rate.

Music As a Focus Tool

In addition to the physical effects, music also diverts your attention. Instead of getting caught up in your thoughts or incessant mind chatter, music absorbs your attention and forces you to focus on something else. So the next time you're feeling stressed, turn on some classical music or a song that you love. Lie down and listen or even dance it out.

Keep a Journal

Getting your thoughts and frustrations out on paper has a proven positive effect on stress levels. You can also use your journal to create daily gratitude lists. Writing down just three things you're grateful for every day will help you further reduce your stress by reminding you of the positive things in your life. They don't have to be big things. In fact, taking stock of the little things in your life will help you appreciate your day-to-day experiences even more. You can write down things like "I'm grateful that I have a bed to sleep in" or "I'm grateful for this cup of coffee." Try to choose different things every day, and you'll see how much you really have to be thankful for—even things that you might not have paid much attention to before.

Journaling is also helpful for keeping track of your emotions and how those emotions affect your eating habits. Write down how you feel each day and what you're eating. When you look back at the pages, you'll be able to recognize how your emotions connect with food (the amount and types that you're eating) and focus on breaking negative behavior patterns that you might not have been aware of otherwise.

Draw Strength from Friends

Studies show that close human bonds are essential to both your physical and mental health, and that social isolation can lead to increased levels of cortisol. Human touch actually stimulates your vagus nerve (one of the nerves that connects your brain to your body), relaxing your nervous system and shutting down your stress response. Touch also increases the release of oxytocin (a hormone linked to feelings of relaxation, trust, and mental stability)—sometimes referred to as the *love hormone*—and reduces the release of cortisol.

Face-to-face contact is best, so find as much time to connect with your loved ones as possible. Surround yourself with supportive people who want to see you succeed in your goals; avoid people who are combative or whom you don't get along with. Tense relationships can increase cortisol levels.

Ease Into Your Fast

If you're new to intermittent fasting or you're used to eating five or six small meals or constantly grazing throughout the day, it can be a big transition to jump right into fasting. You don't have to make a complete change overnight; in fact, you may be more successful if you slowly ease yourself into it.

Start by transitioning from five or six small meals throughout the day to three normal-sized, timed meals. You don't have to eat within a certain window of time yet; just get your body used to the habit and the structure of the three-meal schedule. This will also require you to eliminate snacking throughout the day. Snacking isn't forbidden when you're intermittent fasting, but it can be helpful to eliminate snacks during the beginning stages when you're adjusting. As your body gets used to fasting, you can incorporate snacks during the day as long as you eat them during your feeding window.

Choose a Meal to Skip

Once you've gotten the hang of a three-meal schedule, choose one meal to skip and commit to skipping it each day for a couple of weeks. Don't spend too much time thinking about which meal to skip; you can switch meals later if it works better for you or your schedule. The point is to get your body used to going without food for an extended period of time. Sometimes the hardest part of fasting is training your mind to accept the thought of skipping meals, so this will get you used to that idea.

Work Your Way Up to Your Goal

Once you've gotten the hang of skipping meals and you've chosen which eating plan you're going to follow, slowly work your way up to the ultimate fasting goal. For example, if you're going to follow the 16/8 method and you've decided that your eating window is going to fall between eleven a.m. and seven p.m., but you normally eat breakfast at seven thirty a.m., start by pushing breakfast back to eight thirty a.m. for a couple of days. Then when you're used to the later breakfast, push it back another hour, and then another hour in a few more days until your body is comfortable with waiting until eleven a.m. to eat. Gradually pushing back your eating times won't just help ease you into the fast mentally; it may also help prevent or decrease some of the initial physical symptoms that can occur during the beginning stages of intermittent fasting.

Figure Out Your Eating Plan

The next steps are to figure out what type of eating plan you're going to follow and to find some new and delicious recipes to incorporate into your plan. Fancy, intricate recipes are always tempting—and can be a great treat on the weekends—but in the initial stages of your new fasting plan, it will be easier to keep things simple.

When you're just starting out with intermittent fasting, it's also helpful to scale back on your workout routine. In the very beginning stages of fasting, you may be low on energy and motivation. That's perfectly normal. Instead of engaging in any high-intensity exercises, keep your workouts light. You can resume your workout routine in a couple of weeks when your body has adjusted.

2

Understanding Fasting

Intermittent fasting means changing your approach to your body: what you put into it and how you think about it. It means developing the mental discipline to follow a new lifestyle and to change—often radically—the way you consider what you eat and drink. The better you understand what fasting is all about, the more benefits you'll derive from it. Here we consider some of the things you can anticipate when you start intermittent fasting.

Getting Your Mind Ready

As with any lifestyle change, intermittent fasting may be difficult at first. You may experience some irritability or a drop in energy. You may feel really hungry and have a hard time sticking to your plan. Or you might feel great right off the bat, experiencing positive results immediately and feeling energized and motivated by your new lifestyle. It depends on your body. However, there are some things that are likely to occur as you adjust to your new routine. When you know what to expect and you have some tools ready to cope with any challenges that may arise, your chances for long-term success are much greater.

Consider these popular quotes: "Your mind will quit a thousand times before your body will" and "Your body can stand almost anything. It's your mind you have to convince." The general message behind both of these powerful sayings is that often when you give up, it's not because you've actually reached your physical limit; it's because you've reached your mental limit. In other words, your mind convinces you that your body can't physically handle a challenge, even though it actually can.

Overcoming Negativity

Your brain has a tendency to react more strongly to negative things than it does to positive things. This phenomenon is called the *negativity bias*—and it can be extremely powerful. The biological purpose of the negativity bias is to protect you from possible threats, but in modern times, threats like those faced by your ancestors are fewer and farther between. As a result, you don't need this negativity bias as often, because it's not as helpful as it once was. In fact, this bias makes it harder for you to be present and calm because you're always on alert and anticipating a negative event instead of appreciating the moment. The good news is that you can actually retrain your brain so that it doesn't revert to the negativity bias as easily.

Think Positively

Positive thinking and affirmations are not just New Age trends: they're powerful tools that can actually rewire the neurons in your brain—a concept known as *neuroplasticity*. When you regularly engage in positive thinking and repeat positive affirmations, it makes it easier for your brain to respond more positively to things rather than immediately resorting to its natural negativity bias. And the more you practice, the easier it becomes for your brain to think positively.

Be Aware of the Negative Voice

When you're starting out with intermittent fasting, your subconscious mind will resist the change and will do all it can to get you to resort back to your old routine. When you know this, it's easier to become aware of negative thought patterns and unconstructive self-talk. You may find yourself thinking things like, "This is way too hard," "I'm starving," or "A small snack outside of my fasting window won't hurt." These thoughts are all indications that your negativity bias is running the show. When your mind starts to tell you that it's too hard, recognize that it is this bias talking and respond by saying something like "I'm stronger than my thoughts. I can and will meet my goals."

Focus On the Big Picture

In addition to regularly practicing positive affirmations and changing your negative self-talk, you can also shut your negativity bias down by focusing on the bigger picture. Figure out your main reasons for fasting. Lose weight? Gain more mental clarity and energy? Balance your blood sugar levels? Keep your brain healthy? Whatever your reasons are, write them on a piece of paper or sticky notes and keep them somewhere you will see them frequently, like on the refrigerator. When you feel these negative thoughts start to creep in, read the notes and remember your main goals and why you started in the first place. This can help you see the bigger picture, which will get you through any little speed bumps along the way.

Find Mental Clarity

Once you get past the initial stages of intermittent fasting, it's likely that you'll notice some major changes. Not only will your negative self-talk and negativity bias diminish, but you'll also experience more mental clarity. Intermittent fasting tends to lift brain fog and make concentration easier. You may find that simple tasks become easier and that you're able to focus on your work more. You may also experience less "monkey mind"—intrusive, rapid thoughts that distract you from the task at hand and interfere with your productivity. You may notice your productivity and energy levels increasing. Your memory may feel sharper, and retaining new information may become easier than it was before. You may also notice a stabilization in your moods and emotions—even less anxiety and a more cheerful disposition.

Yes, You're Going to Be Hungry

It's impossible to say exactly how your body will feel during the initial stages of intermittent fasting since everyone is different and you may respond differently from someone else. However, there are a few things that commonly occur in most people when starting intermittent fasting. If you're used to eating five or six times per day, you may experience these effects to a greater degree than if you already eat three meals a day with minimal snacking.

As your body adjusts to intermittent fasting, it's normal to feel increased hunger and cravings. Often this is mental or emotional hunger rather than physical hunger. You may also experience headaches, low energy, and irritability. It's possible to feel a little dizzy, weak, or light-headed upon standing. The severity of these symptoms can vary based on several factors, including your previous eating habits, but they shouldn't be extremely intrusive, and they should diminish within a week or so.

Your Body Will Stabilize

After the initial adjustment period, your blood sugar and insulin levels start to stabilize and you'll begin to reap the benefits of intermittent fasting. One of the first things you'll likely notice is increased energy. You may feel a sustained energy throughout the day; instead of feeling awake and productive in the morning but then being hit with that dreaded afternoon slump around two or three p.m., you'll feel constant energy. This is because your blood sugar isn't spiking and dropping like it does when you eat several meals over the course of the entire day.

Say Goodbye to Puffiness

You may experience a decrease in inflammation, so any puffiness in your face, skin, hands, or feet may start to diminish. Chronic aches and pains that are a regular part of your day may reduce or go away completely. Then you might start to notice that you're dropping a few extra pounds, that you're falling asleep easier, and that the quality of your sleep is better. You'll toss and turn less at night, and as a result you'll wake up feeling refreshed and rested instead of groggy and disoriented. If you're exercising regularly, you might also find it easier to get through your workouts.

The Psychology of Hunger

Hunger is tricky because, on one hand, there's true, physiological hunger; on the other hand, there's mental hunger. Put simply, physical hunger occurs when your stomach is empty. You may feel the physical emptiness in your stomach along with a weakness or a dip in energy. Psychological hunger is the result of a desire to eat out of habit or boredom or because of external cues. While you may do these things subconsciously, when you become aware of them, you can change how they affect you. Instead of mindlessly eating because you're at a social event or your significant other is hungry, pay attention to how you really feel. Are you truly hungry, or are you just tempted by one of these cues? If it's the latter, you can either change your environment or use one of a few helpful techniques provided in this chapter to curb your hunger.

Write It Down

A good way to keep track of changes is to write down any symptoms you feel before starting your intermittent fasting plan. Try to dig deep and be really comprehensive, even listing things that you've dealt with for a long time or that you think have nothing to do with your eating habits. After you've been fasting for a couple of weeks, go back and rewrite your list and compare the two lists. Rewrite your list every couple of weeks after that. This can help you track improvements that you may not even be expecting, and it's likely that you'll be pleasantly surprised.

Hunger Cues

Hunger cues tempt us to eat, even when we're not hungry. There are three kinds of hunger cues: sensory, social, and normative.

An external sensory cue is anything that prompts your desire to eat by targeting your senses. For example, you may smell your favorite meal or see a container full of freshly baked cookies. According to research, exposure to external sensory cues can significantly increase your desire to eat, even when your stomach is full and you're not truly hungry.

Additional Types of Hunger Cues

Food has become a way for people to entertain themselves and others. Going out to eat at a restaurant is now a favorite pastime, and you can rarely go to a party or other event without being offered all types of food. These temptations are social cues. In many of these cases, it's likely that you'll eat even though you're not hungry; often you won't even realize it.

The final type of hunger cues are normative cues; these are things like portion size or plate size, which affect the amount of food you eat. You may not even realize that you're being affected by these things, but research shows that when you use larger plates, you tend to serve yourself more and, as a result, you eat more.

Drink Lots of Water

During your fasting periods (and in general), water should be your best friend. You've probably heard that thirst is often mistaken for hunger, so staying hydrated can help diminish any false hunger signals. Right when you wake up, drink 8 ounces of water. You can prepare by having a glass of water on your nightstand when you go to sleep. Regularly sip water throughout the day and make sure to drink at least half of your body weight in ounces each day. If you exercise a lot or lose sweat in other ways, you may need to drink even more than that. You'll also need to add an extra glass of water for every cup of coffee or other diuretic you drink, so keep that in mind. The more hydrated you are, the less likely you'll experience false hunger signals.

Stay Busy

How many times have you thought you were hungry, but it turned out you were just bored? One minute you're sitting around watching television, and the next minute you're scouring through the pantry for something to snack on. Then, before you know it, an entire bag of chips is empty and you don't even know how it happened.

The best way to avoid this mindless snacking is to keep yourself—and your hands—occupied. Fill your schedule with fun and friends. Do creative projects or immerse yourself fully in work. If you feel boredom creeping in and you're tempted to eat just for the sake of eating, call a friend or a go for a walk around the neighborhood.

Relieve Stress

Stress is a major problem throughout the world. Approximately 77 percent of people in the US report regularly feeling physical symptoms caused by stress, and 33 percent of those people say they are living with extreme stress. Stress can lead not only to weight gain, but also heart disease, diabetes, headaches, depression, anxiety, and gastro-intestinal problems.

One of the immediate ways stress contributes to weight gain is by tempting you to reach for comfort foods—like pizza or ice cream—that you may not crave when your stress levels are more under control. You've most likely heard of emotional eating. Although some people tend to lose their appetite under high stress, many have an increased appetite for foods that are not conducive to a healthy lifestyle.

Stress Management and Hunger

To avoid the dangers of stress-eating, you'll want to find ways to manage your stress. Stress management is especially helpful in keeping hunger cues at bay. Once your stress levels are under control, you'll be able to focus your attention on your eating plan and following the steps to help you reach your goals.

Get Enough Sleep

The importance of sleep cannot be overstated—not just for staving off hunger but for your health in general. Sleep is nourishing and restorative, and when you don't get enough of it, it can completely throw you off in all areas of your life. When you're stressed out, it's easy to skimp out on sleeping in favor of trying to knock a couple more things off of your to-do list, but don't do it! Sleep time is when your brain and body repair and recharge, and it is vital to managing your stress levels and your hunger hormones. Sleep also contributes to improved mood and energy levels, an increased ability to concentrate, and more willpower—which is extremely important in the beginning stages of intermittent fasting.

Ghrelin and Leptin

There are two major hormones—ghrelin and leptin—involved in the hunger response. Ghrelin is the hunger hormone, and when it is released into your body, it tells your brain, "Hey, you're hungry; let's eat." Leptin is the satiation hormone, and it says, "Okay, you're satisfied now. You can stop eating." When you're sleep-deprived, the amount of ghrelin your body produces increases, while the amount of leptin it produces decreases. As a result, your body is constantly telling you that you're hungry and rarely, if ever, telling you that you're satisfied. In addition to this hormonal imbalance, your metabolism slows down when you're sleep-deprived, so you're not as efficiently burning off the food you're eating. For all these reasons, always prioritize sleep.

Stay Focused

The most important thing you can do to ensure your success with intermittent fasting is to have a plan. The first step is to determine which type of fasting you're going to do. Once you've determined the type of fasting, make a schedule. Are you going to fast every day? What times will you fast and what times will you feed? After you've developed your time line, another critical component is determining what you're going to eat when it's time to enter your fed state. Are you going to follow a specific dietary regimen (like the ketogenic diet or Paleo diet) or are you going to stick to a basic clean-eating plan with no real "rules"?

Eliminate Triggers

Look for things that trigger your psychological hunger—and then avoid those things. Up until now, you may have been on autopilot when it comes to eating. You haven't really been paying attention to what is going on around you or what is influencing the amount or the types of food you eat. For example, do you have a significant other who eats twice as much as you do? Do you keep your favorite snacks in the pantry or refrigerator within sight every time you open the doors? Do you schedule social events around food? What kinds of restaurants are you choosing for these events, or what kinds of dishes are you and your friends making?

Figuring out the things that trigger you to eat more—or to choose unhealthy foods—will go a long way not only in maintaining intermittent fasting as a lifestyle but also in preserving your health. Surround yourself with people who support your lifestyle changes and stay away from—or limit time with—people who might sabotage your efforts.

Design Your Meal Plan

First you'll need to design your meal plan. You can plan out a few days, a week, or even the entire month. Find simple recipes and write down everything you'll be eating and at what time. When you're first starting with intermittent fasting and meal planning, the excitement may tempt you to look for fancy, new recipes or a lot of variety, but when you're in the initial stages of a new lifestyle change, one of the most beneficial things you can do is stick to the basics and not overcomplicate things.

Go with What You Know

Stick to foods that you're already familiar with and recipes that won't take too long to prepare or that require you to learn new kitchen skills or buy new kitchen tools. There will be plenty of time for you to try new things after you get used to the basics and your body and mind adjust to the changes. The point of meal prepping is to make you feel less overwhelmed, not to add any unnecessary stress.

There are online meal planners and trackers as well as phone apps that you can use to keep track of your meals, but you don't need any fancy tools or software if technology isn't your thing. You can keep it simple by recording everything in a notebook.

Draw Up a Grocery List

Once you've gotten your recipes together and your meal plan written out, it's time to figure out what you need. Check your refrigerator and your pantry prior to writing your grocery list so you don't purchase things you already have. After you've compiled a list of things you have on hand, write out a grocery list of the remaining items you'll need to complete your recipes and your meals for the week (or for whatever length of time you've chosen).

You can save even more time by organizing your grocery list based on where items are found in the supermarket. You can list all meats together, all produce items together, and all refrigerated items together. If you need to go to different stores for any deals or any specialty items, organize your lists by store.

Prep Your Meals

Once you've gotten the basics down, prepping your meals can help keep you on track and prevent you from reaching for an unhealthy meal in times of hunger. Research shows that people who prepare their meals ahead of time experience greater success with their health and nutrition goals and also save time and money in the long run. As you get into the groove of intermittent fasting and your new way of eating, you can make adjustments to your meals and your prepping routine.

Getting organized is one of the most vital components of successful meal prep. It may seem daunting or like a waste of time to sit down and organize recipes and write everything out, but it will end up saving you time down the road.

The amount of meals you prepare in advance and the amount of time you spend cooking is completely up to you. Some people spend three or four hours on Sunday prepping meals for the entire week. Others spend a couple of hours on Sunday prepping meals for the next few days and then spend another couple of hours on Wednesday prepping meals for the rest of the week. Regardless of what style of meal prepping you choose, organization is key.

Don't Obsess over the Scale

If weight loss is one of your goals, don't rely solely on the scale. Your actual weight can fluctuate significantly from day to day, and you might not see big changes in the numbers even when your body is going through a massive transformation. You can use the scale as a tool, but take these day-to-day numbers with a grain of salt.

"Before" and "After"

Instead, take "before" and "after" (or "progress") pictures. Down the line, you can compare them side by side to see how your body has changed over time. Pictures can be a really motivating tool because when you see yourself every day, you may not notice the small changes occurring, but when you compare pictures that were taken a month apart, the changes may be significantly more apparent. Don't let any current dissatisfaction with your body stop you from taking "before" pictures. You'll be happy you have them down the road.

Body Measurements

It's helpful to take body measurements. You may start to build more lean muscle mass, especially if you're working out or doing strength training regularly. As your body starts to change, you may not notice too much of a shift on the scale, but your body composition can change dramatically. Measurements can help you track progress by documenting inches lost from different areas of your body.

What to Measure

You'll want to take the following measurements:

- **Bust:** measure all the way around your bust, keeping the measuring tape in line with your nipples.
- **Chest:** measure directly underneath your breasts or pectoral muscles and all the way around your back.
- **Hips:** find the widest area of your hips and measure all the way around.
- **Knees:** measure all the way around directly above the knee while standing up straight.
- **Lower arms:** measure all the way around the fullest part of your lower arm below your elbow.
- **Thighs:** measure all the way around the fullest part of your upper leg while standing up straight.
- **Upper arms:** measure all the way around the fullest part of your upper arm above your elbow.
- **Waist:** find the narrowest part of your waist, usually right below your rib cage, and measure all the way around.

The Tale of the Tape

To properly measure, you'll need a nonstretchable measuring tape. Keep the tape level around your body and parallel to the floor. When you're taking your measurements, wrap the tape around your body as close to your skin as possible, but don't squeeze so tightly that the tape measure cuts into your skin or makes an indentation. It's helpful to have someone else take your measurements for you so you can stand straight; if you don't have someone available, take your measurements in front of a mirror to make sure that you're keeping the tape level and measuring in the correct spots.

Make a list of your measurements in a notebook or in your phone's notepad. Take your measurements every few weeks and record the numbers in the same place every time. As time passes, you can use the measurements to chart your progress.

There Will Be Ups and Downs

Like anything in life, you'll experience ups and downs with intermittent fasting, especially in the very beginning. Don't expect everything to go smoothly right off the bat and don't get caught up in perfection. You're going to slip up: you're going to eat outside of your feeding window sometimes, and that's okay. If you go into it knowing that you're going to put your best foot forward but also understanding that it can take a little while to get used to the transition, you'll be less likely to beat yourself up when things don't go totally according to plan.

Fasting Is Your Friend

The benefits of fasting extend to practically all aspects of your health, both physical and mental. As long as you do it responsibly and carefully, it can help you take control of your body and your well-being. There are many ways of intermittent fasting. You need to choose the method that works best for you and puts you on the road toward achieving your health goals. Sometimes you'll mix and match methods or experiment until you find one that you can commit to.

Fasting and a Healthy Lifestyle

One of the most common reasons people jump into intermittent fasting is weight loss, but that's barely scratching the surface. Intermittent fasting does so much more for your body than helping you shed pounds. It also helps stabilize your blood sugar levels, decease chronic or widespread inflammation, and improve your heart health. Studies have also shown that intermittent fasting may contribute to brain health, helping decrease your risk of developing major brain diseases like Alzheimer's. Finally, it's been suggested by some researchers that it may help with cancer prevention and enhance the effects of chemotherapy for those who are suffering from the disease.

Lose Weight

You've probably heard that if you eat less, you lose more weight—but what if weight loss has less to do with the amount of food you're eating and more to do with the amount of time during which you're eating it? When you hear how intermittent fasting works, you may think, "Well, yeah, if you're eating during a smaller window of time, you'll be eating fewer calories, and that's why you lose weight." That's part of it: in some cases, you'll be eating fewer calories, especially because you'll be cutting out the late-night mindless snacking that can quickly contribute to weight gain. But that's not the whole story. Studies have shown that intermittent fasting can reduce weight and improve metabolism even without an overall calorie restriction.

Drop Visceral Fat

One study published in *Translational Research* found that intermittent fasting can reduce body weight by 3–8 percent in a period of three to twenty-four weeks. The participants in this study also lost 4–7 percent of their waist circumference, which indicates that they lost belly fat, or visceral fat, which is the type of fat thought to be most dangerous to physical heath.

Visceral fat is stored deep inside the abdominal cavity. It lies in close proximity to several vital organs, including the liver, stomach, pancreas, and intestines. Having a lot of visceral fat is more dangerous than having extra subcutaneous fat (the fat that lies just underneath your skin) because visceral fat can affect your hormones and the way your body operates. It's linked to a greater risk of heart disease, cancer, stroke, diabetes, arthritis, obesity, and depression. There's no surefire way to tell if your fat is subcutaneous or visceral, but if you carry a lot of weight around your midsection, it's likely that you have a higher percentage of visceral fat.

Intermittent Fasting and Diets

Studies also show that people who follow dietary plans that allow variability in food choices, like intermittent fasting, are more likely to stick to the diet and maintain weight loss than those who follow a rigid, calorie-controlled diet. Rigid diets are also associated with symptoms of disordered eating and a higher body mass index (a measure of your body fat using weight and height) in nonobese women, while flexible dieting strategies, like intermittent fasting, are not.

Hearing this may be discouraging, especially if you've subscribed to the theory that the way to lose weight is to restrict calories and exercise more—but this is actually good news. You don't have to spend your days counting calories, eating too little, and avoiding healthy fats. There's a better way: intermittent fasting. (Just a note here: fasting works well for some people and not for others. You need to find the best way of losing weight, one that works for you.)

Disproving an Old Myth

The most common and persistent weight-loss theories are "eat less, move more" and "calories in versus calories out." The general principle underlying these theories is that if you take in fewer calories than you burn off, you'll lose weight, but if you look at the statistics, these notions don't add up. For the past twenty years, people have been instructed to follow low-calorie, low-fat diets and to eat five to six small meals each day. Yet during these twenty years, obesity rates have increased substantially. Of course, there's the argument that people simply just aren't putting in the work required to lose weight, but in many cases this isn't true. There are scores of people who exercise regularly and eat "healthily" yet still have nothing to show for it. This is because weight loss isn't that simple—and conventional wisdom has been proven wrong.

The Women's Health Initiative study followed approximately fifty thousand women for a period of almost eight years. During that time, one half of the women followed a low-fat, low-calorie diet and increased their exercise output by 14 percent. This group was classified as the *intervention group*. The second half of the women followed their usual diet and exercise routine. The average difference in weight loss in the intervention group after almost eight years? Less than 2 pounds.

Women and Fasting

There is a commonly held belief that fasting is bad for women, and while this can be true for some women, it's not a blanket statement that can be applied to all women. This theory developed due to the fact that intermittent fasting has the potential to cause a hormonal imbalance in some women if the fasting is not done properly; but when the proper care and precautions are taken, women can fast successfully.

Because women's bodies were physiologically designed to carry babies, women are more sensitive to potential starvation than men. If a woman's body senses any impending starvation, it will respond by increasing the hormones leptin and ghrelin, which work together to control hunger. This hormonal response is the female body's way of protecting a developing fetus, even if a woman is not currently pregnant.

Although it's possible to ignore the hunger signals from ghrelin and leptin, it becomes increasingly difficult, especially as the body revolts and starts to produce more of these hormones. If a woman gives in to the hunger in an unhealthy way—by overeating or consuming unhealthy foods—this can cause a cascade of other hormonal issues involving insulin.

This process can also shut down the reproductive system. If your body thinks it doesn't have enough food to survive, it might shut down the ability to conceive to protect a potential pregnancy. This is why fasting is not recommended during pregnancy or for women who are trying to become pregnant.

The Human Growth Hormone

Human growth hormone, or HGH, is a naturally occurring hormone that's produced by your pituitary gland—a small endocrine gland in your brain that also controls your adrenals and thyroid. When your body releases HGH, the hormone stays in the bloodstream, where the liver converts it into other active growth factors, such as insulin-like growth factor, or IGF-1. These growth factors promote growth in every cell of your body. When you fast, the levels of HGH in your body naturally increase. In fact, some research shows that the levels can increase as much as five times when compared to times you don't fast.

One of the most notable benefits of HGH is its ability to stimulate the synthesis of collagen in both the skeletal muscles and tendons. Muscles and tendons that contain more collagen result in increased muscle strength, which can improve your physical capabilities and exercise performance. Having more muscle mass also increases your basal metabolic rate. This makes your body more efficient at using up calories, even when you're not active. HGH also increases lipolysis—a physiological process during which fat and triglycerides are broken apart and turned into free fatty acids, which are then removed from the body. An increase in lipolysis translates to easier and faster weight loss.

Fasting and Autophagy

Autophagy is a normal physiological process that is involved in cleaning out old or destroyed compounds in the body. Although it sounds a little unnerving, the literal translation of autophagy is "self-eating." It's derived from the Greek words *autos*, which translates to "self," and *phagein*, which means "to eat." The term *autophagy* was coined by Christian de Duve, a Nobel Prize–winning scientist, after a group of researchers noticed an increase in lysosomes (the parts of the cells responsible for breaking down and destroying other compounds) in liver cells after injections of glucagon, the hormone that works in opposition to insulin.

Autophagy plays a key role in maintaining homeostasis—a stable and healthy internal environment—in the body. Your body constantly has proteins and organelles (small, specialized structures in each of your body's cells) that become dysfunctional or die. If allowed to accumulate in the body, these dead tissues can cause cell death, contribute to poor tissue and/or organ function, and even become cancerous. During autophagy, the body marks damaged parts of cells and unused proteins in the body. These damaged parts are sent to the lysosomes, where they're cleared out of the body. This process prevents them from causing harm.

Autophagy and Natural Immunity

There's also evidence that autophagy may play a role in decreasing chronic inflammation and boosting natural immunity. Research shows that subjects who are not capable of inducing autophagy tend to carry more weight, sleep more often, and have higher cholesterol levels and decreased brain function.

Fasting is one of the most effective ways to stimulate autophagy in both the body and the brain because depriving the body of certain nutrients for a set period of time turns the process on. When insulin goes up (after eating), glucagon (the hormone that acts opposite to insulin) goes down. Conversely, when insulin goes down (after a period without food), glucagon goes up. When you fast, glucagon increases, stimulating autophagy.

The 16/8 Method

The 16/8 method of fasting, also known as the *Leangains protocol*, is the most popular type of intermittent fasting. It was originally developed by Martin Berkhan, a nutritional expert and personal trainer who was looking for a way to help his clients build muscle without accumulating fat. When following the 16/8 method, you schedule a sixteen-hour fasting window and an eight-hour feeding window each day. This means that you'll go for sixteen hours without eating anything, fitting all of your meals within a consecutive eight-hour time frame. For example, you may choose a fasting window between seven p.m. and eleven a.m., which means the feeding window would fall between eleven a.m. and seven p.m.

There are no hard rules about the times you must eat, but once you decide on a schedule, you'll want to stick to it every day. Berkhan says that if you don't have a consistent feeding window, it can throw your hormones out of whack and make it even harder to stick to the program because you'll experience more hunger and may not notice any of the positive health benefits. There are also no restrictions on the amount of meals you eat: you can fit breakfast, lunch, dinner, and even some snacks into the eight-hour eating window. Of course, if weight loss is one of your goals, you'll want to be more mindful of your calorie intake.

Drinking While Fasting

During your fasting window, you are allowed to drink water, coffee, and other noncaloric beverages, such as tea or seltzer; however, pay attention to your caffeine intake and be careful not to overdo it. While sipping beverages during your fasting window can help stave off hunger, too much caffeine can leave you anxious, jittery, and dehydrated, especially when your stomach is empty. Caffeine also puts stress on your adrenals, so while your body is adjusting to the added stress of fasting, it's best to keep your coffee intake minimal.

One of the major benefits of the 16/8 method of intermittent fasting is that it's fairly easy to incorporate into your schedule. Since you'll be sleeping for around eight hours of your fast, you have to skip food for only a small portion of your waking hours. Most people can successfully pull off the 16/8 method by not eating after dinner and then skipping breakfast or eating it late in the morning.

Eat Unprocessed Foods

Although there isn't a specific diet you must follow while doing the 16/8 method, Martin Berkhan, who developed the method, recommends that whole, unprocessed foods make up the majority of your calorie intake. You may need to watch carefully for sales and buy in bulk, but unprocessed foods can fit into your meal budget. It just takes a bit of planning. In addition to eating as cleanly as possible, you should incorporate protein as a moderate portion of your calorie intake. On the days you exercise, most of the calories you don't take in from protein should be from carbohydrates. On rest days, fat intake should be higher than carbohydrate intake.

Your Circadian Rhythm

It's helpful to know what your circadian rhythm is and how it affects your body. Also referred to as a *body clock* or a *biological clock*, your circadian rhythm is a twenty-four-hour cycle that regulates many of your body's physiological processes, like sleep and digestion. Your body receives cues from your circadian rhythm about when to go to sleep, when to wake up, and when to eat.

Your circadian rhythm is controlled internally by an area of your brain called the *hypothalamus*, but it's largely affected by external, environmental cues like temperature and light. For example, when it's dark outside, your eyes send a signal to your hypothalamus that it's time to sleep; your hypothalamus sends a message to the pineal gland (in another area of the brain) to release melatonin (a hormone that helps you sleep), and you get tired. When it's light out, the opposite happens. Your eyes send a signal to your hypothalamus, which sends a signal to your pineal gland to decrease the production of melatonin. This dip in melatonin helps wake you up and prepare you for the day.

Your circadian rhythm is also affected by the timing of your meals. In the Paleolithic era, food was available mostly during daylight hours. This is because food needed to be hunted and gathered, and it was easier to do this during the day. Biologically, the human body prefers this cycle and has yet to properly adjust to the changes brought about by the Industrial Revolution and modern conveniences like grocery stores and artificial lighting.

The Warrior Diet

The warrior diet, which was developed by Ori Hofmekler, a member of the Israeli Special Forces, is credited with being the catalyst to other intermittent fasting methods. Hofmekler introduced the warrior diet in 2001 after spending time in the army and studying the behavior and dietary patterns of the warrior societies of Rome and Sparta. He designed the warrior diet based on the belief that it was the natural way to eat before the Industrial Revolution, and that following it could promote both weight loss and increased energy.

The warrior diet takes the 16/8 method one step further by extending the fasting period to closer to twenty hours. While following the warrior diet, you eat only one large meal at night. During the day, you can have light snacks—like berries, yogurt, and whey protein—as well as water, vegetable juices, coffee, and tea. The fasting part of the warrior diet is the "undereating" phase, and the four-hour feeding window is the "overeating" phase.

The undereating phase takes place during the day because the stress of less food triggers the sympathetic nervous system's fight-or-flight response. As a result, you experience a boost in energy, a rise in adrenaline (which promotes alertness), and an increase in fat burning. The overeating phase takes place at night because the goal during this phase is to do the opposite of the undereating phase by triggering the parasympathetic nervous system's rest-and-digest response. When the body is in rest-and-digest mode, it promotes calmness and relaxation, improves digestion, and helps the body recuperate from the stresses of the day. When the body is relaxed, it's also able to use the nutrients you take in more efficiently.

Restrictions on Food Combinations

Unlike other fasting methods, which don't specify exactly what types of food to eat during your feeding period, the warrior diet restricts certain combinations of food. For example, while following the warrior diet, you can combine protein and vegetables but must avoid combining nuts and fruits, grains and fruits, protein and grains, and alcohol and starch. The theory behind this is that your body is able to digest certain combinations of foods better than others. Combining protein and vegetables is easy on digestion, while combining protein with grains makes digestion more difficult.

During your four-hour eating window, you'll start by eating non-starchy vegetables, protein, and fat. Once that settles, you can add in some carbohydrates if you're still hungry. The theory behind this is that eating in this pattern can optimize hormone production and the way your body burns fat during the day.

The warrior diet doesn't just focus on intermittent fasting, though; the true warrior diet also requires regular exercise during your fasted state. According to research, you can burn up to 20 percent more fat when you exercise in a fasted state. The theory is that high insulin levels can suppress the way your body metabolizes fat. When you fast, your insulin levels drop. If you activate your metabolism by exercising when insulin levels are low, you'll be able to burn more fat.

Eat Stop Eat Method

Instead of fasting every day, the Eat Stop Eat method involves incorporating a twenty-four-hour fast for either one or two days per week and then eating normally on the other five or six days. With the Eat Stop Eat method, you choose the days and times of your fasts, but you must make sure that you're not eating for a full twenty-four hours. For example, your schedule may be to eat normally Tuesday through Sunday but to fast from Sunday night at eight p.m. to Monday night at eight p.m. Like with the 16/8 method, you cannot eat any food during your fasting windows, but you're allowed to drink calorie-free beverages. When your fast is over, you go back to eating normally.

Brad Pilon, founder of the Eat Stop Eat method, believes that you're taught from a young age that you have to eat at certain times, and this idea can put a strain on you and on how you feel about eating in general. He defines intermittent fasting as "the ability to practice patience when it comes to the act of eating—a conscious polite restraint when it comes to food intake." His philosophy is that "we do not have to eat all the time; therefore we are free to choose when we eat."

Because most of the focus on the Eat Stop Eat method is on meal timing, Pilon doesn't define any foods as forbidden or off-limits. You don't have to count calories or restrict your diet, and not doing either makes it easier to follow on feeding days, but if you want optimal results or your goal is to lose weight, you'll have to make smart choices when it comes to what you're eating.

The 5:2 Method

The 5:2 method, also called the *5:2 fast diet* and the *fast diet*, was made popular by Michael Mosley, a British physician and journalist. Like the Eat Stop Eat method, the 5:2 method involves fasting only on certain days of the week. With this method of fasting, you don't ever completely abstain from eating: you eat normally on five days of the week and then restrict calories to 500–600 per day on the other two days of the week.

For example, while following the 5:2 method, you may eat normally on Monday, Wednesday, Thursday, Saturday, and Sunday but restrict calories on Tuesday and Friday. You choose the days of the week you fast, but you must incorporate a nonfasting day in between your fasting days.

What "normal" eating is for you depends on your height, weight, sex, and activity levels, as well as your weight goals. There are several free online calculators (you can search "online calorie calculator" to find many options) that let you type in your statistics and goals and get a recommendation on how many calories you should be eating on your "normal" days.

Alternate-Day Fasting

There are two ways to do alternate-day fasting. The first—and less common—way is to alternate days of eating normally with days of complete fasting. This means that you would eat normally on Monday, completely abstain from food Tuesday, eat normally on Wednesday, completely abstain from food on Thursday, and so on. The second way involves modified fasting. When you follow the modified alternate-day fasting, you eat normally every other day and eat approximately one-fifth of your normal calories on the remaining days. For a typical diet of 2,000–2,500 calories per day, this means that you would eat 400–500 calories on your modified fasting days. The goal is to cut calories by 20–35 percent per week. Research shows that people are able to stick with alternate-day fasting much easier than traditional low-calorie diets that require calorie restriction on every day of the week.

Like many of the other methods of fasting, you're allowed to drink as many calorie-free beverages as you want during your fasting time. If you choose to follow the modified fasting version, there are no restrictions about what times you consume your calories during the day. You can have one large meal during the day or spread mini meals or snacks out throughout the entire day

Spontaneous Fasting

Unlike the other types of fasting, which are more rigid in their specific time frames, spontaneous fasting involves skipping meals spontaneously. For example, if you're not hungry in the morning, skip breakfast and eat only lunch and dinner. Or, if you're too busy to eat lunch, skip it.

The key with spontaneous fasting, though, is in making sure that you're eating healthy foods for the meals that you don't skip. Of course, this is important with all types of fasting, but it can be especially important with spontaneous fasting since there's less structure and the temptation to overeat unhealthy foods may be higher.

Getting Your Feet Wet

Spontaneous fasting is a good way to get your feet wet with intermittent fasting. You can skip a meal here or there to get your body used to going an extended period of time without eating, then slowly transition to one of the other fasting plans. Or, if it works for you, you can stick with the spontaneous fasting indefinitely. Another benefit to spontaneous fasting is that it's easy to fit into your schedule because you can skip meals when it's convenient for you and eat meals when you have time to prepare something healthy.

Extended Fasting

Although extended fasting belongs in a class of its own, it's important to know the difference between it and the other types of intermittent fasting. Extended fasting is any type of fast that lasts for more than twenty-four hours. Often, extended fasting can last a week, and many of these extended fasts involve consuming only water.

These types of fasts are more common in medical and hospital settings and are usually done when the body needs to undergo significant healing or when the ability to eat is compromised. You should not start an extended fast without the recommendation and supervision of a medical professional.

Other Ways You Can Extend Autophagy

Although fasting is the most effective way to stimulate autophagy, you can also kick on this process through exercise and by following a ketogenic diet. This is why many people who fast decide to follow a ketogenic diet as well: it's a double whammy for cellular cleansing. The ketogenic diet helps stimulate autophagy by tricking the body into thinking it's going without food, so the same metabolic changes are seen. When you drastically lower carbohydrates, it forces your body to turn to using fat as an energy source instead. Doing this also keeps insulin levels low and glucagon levels high—a must for getting autophagy started.

Exercise is another effective way to stimulate autophagy, and because of this, regular exercise has been shown to kill cancerous cells. One study published in *Autophagy* found that autophagy increases significantly after jogging for thirty minutes on a treadmill and continues increasing up to eighty total minutes of exercise, when it begins to level out. The effect is seen to a greater degree with intense exercise.

Choosing the Best Plan for You

There are many different variations for intermittent fasting because there is no one-size-fits-all approach. The plan that works best for you may not be the plan that works best for your neighbor and vice versa. To decide which intermittent fasting type is best for you, you'll have to ask yourself a series of questions.

One of the most important things to do is figure out which type of plan works best with your schedule. Of course, it's possible to re-arrange your schedule around your new eating plan—and for some people this may be necessary—but you're more likely to stick to a new routine if it falls somewhat easily into your life. For many people, the 16/8 method is the plan that makes most sense with their schedule because most of the fasting time occurs overnight. However, if you're not on a typical schedule or you have longer work hours and you have to be up for a longer portion of the day, this may not work as well for you. For example, if you don't work a typical Monday through Friday job and you have Monday and Thursday off instead, you may find that the 5:2 method works better for your schedule because you can eat normally while you're at work and then use your days off for your fasting days.

What Plan Will You Stick To?

Sometimes, just figuring out which plan works best with your schedule isn't enough. In order to experience any lasting benefits of intermittent fasting, you'll have to actually stick to it. You'll need to find a plan that fits into your schedule. If the 16/8 method seems best in theory but you know you would have a hard time going for sixteen hours without food, then maybe a modified alternate-day fasting protocol is better for you.

Don't put too much pressure on yourself to be perfect or to follow a certain protocol down to the letter, especially at first. Adjusting to intermittent fasting can take some time, especially if you're used to eating small meals all day long. Be gentle with yourself and give yourself time to adapt and adjust.

Mix and Match

You can use the outlined methods to create your own protocol, or you can even mix up the protocols as you go. For example, you can follow the basics of the 16/8 method but fast for thirteen to fourteen hours instead of sixteen. You can use Eat Stop Eat as a template but fast for sixteen or eighteen hours for a couple days each week until you can work your way up to a twenty-four-hour fast. Remember, the only way any of these methods will work is if you're able to stick to them. Modifying one of the protocols so that you can stick to it for the long haul is better than trying to follow a protocol exactly as written and quitting after a couple of weeks because you're so frustrated.

Exercise While Fasting

There's a long-standing debate in the fitness world about whether it's better to work out on an empty stomach (a fasted state) or a full stomach (a fed state). The answer is that it depends on the intensity of your exercise. There are many benefits to exercising in a fasted state, but if you're an endurance athlete or engaging in high-intensity exercise, working out after eating may be better for you.

Getting Enough Energy

When you exercise, your body demands an increased amount of energy. First, your body will turn for fuel to glucose in the blood. When that runs out, it starts burning glycogen—the form of glucose that's stored in the liver. In general, your liver stores enough glycogen to sustain your body's energy needs for twenty-four hours in the absence of food; however, the increased energy demand that exercise puts on the body will result in a faster depletion of glycogen. The amount of glycogen that gets used up depends on the duration and the intensity of the exercise you're doing.

Once glycogen is depleted, your body switches from burning carbohydrates for energy to burning stored fat. Your body's ability to burn fat is controlled by your sympathetic nervous system, which is turned on by both fasting and exercise. When you combine the two, it maximizes the physiological processes that break down fat for energy. Unlike glycogen, which is only stored in limited amounts, fat can be stored in your body in unlimited amounts, so you never run out. Your muscles will eventually adapt to using whatever energy source you give them.

The Hormonal Benefits of Fasted Exercise

In addition to increasing fat burn, exercising on an empty stomach has also been shown to optimize health by improving levels of two specific hormones: insulin and growth hormone.

Research shows that fasted exercise may have a positive effect on insulin sensitivity (the way the body responds to insulin). When you eat too much, your blood sugar spikes, and as a result your body is exposed to a constant barrage of insulin. Over time this can cause an insulin overload that weakens the way your cells respond to the hormone. By exercising in a fasted state, you're not only giving your body a break from releasing insulin into the blood but you're also burning up any excess insulin that your body may have. When your body responds to insulin in a healthy way, it makes it easier to lose fat and improves blood flow to muscles, making it easier to build muscles. Fasted exercise increases the production of growth hormone, which not only helps burn fat and increase muscle tissue but also improves bone health.

High-Intensity Exercise

On the days when you want to do high-intensity exercise like high-intensity interval training (HIIT)—a type of workout where you alternate short bursts of high-intensity exercise with longer periods of lower-intensity exercise—or strength training, schedule your training close to a meal. When you exercise in a fed state, you provide your body with glucose and glycogen to push you through your workouts. This will prevent muscle loss and low blood sugar levels.

A good way to gauge the intensity of your workout is the talk test. During a low-intensity workout, you should be able to carry on a conversation fairly easily. When the exercise is high-intensity, you should be able to comfortably say only a few words at a time. If you can't talk at all during your workout without losing your breath, you're exercising too hard.

Tips for Exercise

Regular exercise is a vital component to staying healthy, so while it can take some extra planning to get into the proper groove when you're intermittent fasting, it's important that you keep a regular routine. It always comes back to listening to your body's specific needs.

If you're looking to build some serious muscle, schedule all strength-training sessions between two meals. Your muscles need amino acids to repair themselves and grow after weight lifting, so if adding muscle is your goal, eat a protein-rich meal an hour before your strength-training session and another protein-rich meal sixty to ninety minutes after your workout is over. According to the Academy of Nutrition and Dietetics, you should aim for 20–30 grams of high-quality protein per meal.

Keep in mind that many people easily eat well over their recommended protein needs each day, so you don't have to go crazy. To give you some perspective, a 6-ounce chicken breast contains 52 grams of protein.

Benefits, Risks, and Concerns
of Intermittent Fasting

Before beginning a regimen of intermittent fasting, you should clearly understand not only what it can do to help you but also what some of the risks are. There are many myths about fasting, and you should know what's true and what's not. To help you with this, we'll examine how fasting affects many of the body's systems and what kind of fasting will work best for you depending on your current health patterns.

Improve Your Metabolism

Many people believe that the solution to keeping your metabolism at peak condition is to eat small meals frequently. That's why you hear the advice that it's better to eat five or six small meals throughout the day than to eat two or three larger meals. But the only way your body will enter a true starvation mode (and really damage your metabolism) is if you go a prolonged period of time—days or weeks, as opposed to hours—without eating. If the body went into starvation mode within hours, it would be highly disadvantageous to the survival of the human species. In Paleolithic times, a decrease in metabolism would also mean a decrease in energy, which would make it harder to hunt and gather food. If hunters and gatherers couldn't obtain food, metabolism would drop even more and energy would continue to plummet, eventually leading to an inability to survive.

Studies show that intermittent fasting doesn't inhibit your ability to burn off extra calories and fat: it actually has the opposite effect on your metabolic rate. According to research published in *The American Journal of Clinical Nutrition* and *The American Journal of Physiology*, the number of calories you burn at rest—also called your basal metabolic rate (or BMR)—actually increases by a significant amount when you incorporate short-term fasting. The reason for this is that when you enter a fasted state, the levels of norepinephrine—a stress hormone and neurotransmitter—in your blood decrease. This stimulates your metabolism and signals your body to break down excess body fat.

Balance Your Insulin and Glucose

Your body obtains energy from three main sources that are known as *macronutrients*: carbohydrates, fat, and protein—in that order. The ingestion of these macronutrients causes a rise in both glucose and insulin, but the degree at which these levels rise differs based on which one you are eating and how much of it you are eating.

Carbohydrates, especially refined carbohydrates and simple sugars, cause the most substantial increases in both glucose and insulin, whereas fat and protein cause more moderate increases. This is significant because the rises in blood sugar and insulin affect the way you use the sugar and the hormone. The way your body responds to insulin says a lot about your ability to lose weight and your health in general.

One of insulin's main jobs is to move glucose from your bloodstream into your cells, where it's used as energy, or to move it to the liver, where it's converted to glycogen and stored for later use. If you are resistant to insulin, your body doesn't respond to normal amounts of insulin properly, and instead of moving to your cells, glucose and insulin remain in the bloodstream. When glucose and insulin stay floating in your blood, the pancreas releases even more insulin in an effort to lower your glucose (blood sugar) levels. High insulin levels are connected to a reduced ability to burn fat—in other words, difficulty losing weight. But what causes insulin resistance and how can you reverse it? Fasting.

Insulin Resistance

Statistics show that approximately sixty to seventy million adults are affected by insulin resistance. If not corrected, insulin resistance can destroy the beta cells (the cells responsible for producing and releasing insulin) in the pancreas and contribute to the development of pre-diabetes and diabetes. The American Diabetes Association (ADA) estimates that 70 percent of those with insulin resistance will go on to develop type 2 diabetes if significant lifestyle changes aren't made.

The way to help correct insulin resistance is to lower the amount of insulin that your body is producing—and you can do this by eating less. When you eat, the levels of glucose and insulin in your body rise. As a result, your body starts burning off glucose for energy instead of fat. When you don't eat, glucose and insulin levels stay lower, and your body turns to stored fat for energy—ultimately resulting in weight loss.

Fight Against Prediabetes and Diabetes

According to the 2017 National Diabetes Statistics Report released by the Centers for Disease Control and Prevention, approximately 30.3 million Americans are currently living with diabetes, and 7.2 million of them are undiagnosed cases. Another 84.1 million adults (almost 34 percent of the adult US population) are living with prediabetes.

When you fast and teach your body to burn fat for energy instead of glucose, it not only lowers insulin and blood sugar levels but also improves insulin sensitivity. Balanced blood sugar levels are also associated with:

- Improved fasting blood glucose (blood sugar levels after going twelve hours without eating)
- Improved postprandial blood glucose (blood sugar levels after eating a meal)
- Reduced glucose variability (drastic increases and dips in blood sugar levels)

Reduced glucose variability is especially notable when it comes to concerns with hunger. When you get hungry after a short period of time without food, it's often because your blood sugar dips dramatically after an increase. This is because your pancreas releases a rush of insulin in response to the presence of glucose in your blood. When the insulin rushes into your blood and carries the glucose into your cells, it results in a decrease in blood sugar. This decrease is the cause of hunger and any uncomfortable symptoms that come with it. The greater the initial spike in blood sugar, the greater the resulting dip will be.

Improve Your Blood Sugar Regulation

When you fast, there are no rapid increases in blood sugar, which means there are no dramatic decreases either. As a result, you'll experience less hunger, and you'll avoid the other symptoms of low blood sugar, which include:

- Anxiety
- Blurred vision
- Confusion
- Dizziness or light-headedness
- Dry mouth
- Fatigue
- Headache
- Increased sweating
- Irritability
- Shakiness

Of course, it may take some time for your body to adjust to your new lifestyle and for your blood sugar levels to regulate. Because of this, you may experience some symptoms of low blood sugar when you first start your fasting regimen.

Reduce Chronic Inflammation

Your body experiences chronic inflammation in response to a prolonged threat. The trouble is that the threat is not often obvious. You may experience chronic inflammation in response to a pathogen that the body cannot break down, such as a stubborn virus that remains in your system, or an overactive immune response from an undiagnosed food sensitivity. Chronic inflammation can also arise from prolonged, unmanaged stress. Whatever the cause, chronic inflammation can be dangerous to your health. Unlike acute inflammation, which typically goes away after a few days, chronic inflammation can last from several months to a number of years. If chronic inflammation is left untreated, it can cause thickening and scarring of connective tissue and even result in tissue death. Some conditions associated with chronic inflammation include:

- Autoimmune diseases
- Cancer
- Chronic respiratory diseases, like asthma
- Diabetes
- Heart disease
- Neurological diseases
- Obesity
- Stroke
- Ulcerative colitis and Crohn's disease

Fasting can help reduce chronic inflammation. Leukotrienes are biologically active molecules that are formed by leukocytes (a type of white blood cell.) They are pro-inflammatory and play a major role in asthma attacks, allergic diseases, and anaphylaxis, which is a severe, potentially fatal allergic reaction. Leukotrienes are also involved in a wide variety of other diseases. While small amounts of leukotrienes are helpful for acute inflammation, higher levels contribute to chronic inflammation.

Block Inflammasomes

Through separate studies, researchers at Yale University found that when you fast, your body produces a compound that can block the part of the immune system that's involved in various inflammatory disorders. These blocked receptors and sensors, known as *inflammasomes*, are connected to a number of different inflammatory disorders. Research shows that inflammasomes are at least partly responsible for the development and progression of metabolic diseases, like diabetes and nonalcoholic fatty liver disease, and neurodegenerative diseases, like Parkinson's disease, dementia, and Huntington's disease.

When you fast, your body produces a compound called beta-hydroxybutyrate (BHB). BHB acts directly on a certain inflammasome called NLRP3, shutting off the inflammatory response and reducing the negative effects of chronic inflammation on the body.

Help Your Heart Health

In the United States, heart disease is the leading cause of death for both men and women. Every year, approximately 610,000 deaths (which averages out to about one in four deaths) are attributed to heart disease. The American Heart Association asserts that the biggest contributor to these statistics is the lack of commitment to a heart-healthy lifestyle. In other words, many cases of heart disease develop due to risk factors that you can control. One of these major risk factors is your diet.

Although medical experts agree that a heart-healthy lifestyle can help lower your risk of heart disease, there is some disagreement about what that lifestyle actually entails. There is a pervasive myth that one of the best things you can do for your heart is follow a low-fat, low-cholesterol diet, even though research has disproven this time and time again.

Understand Cholesterol

Cholesterol has developed a really bad reputation, but the lipoprotein—as cholesterol is physiologically classified—is largely misunderstood. Cholesterol performs three major functions in your body, and without it, you wouldn't be able to survive. It's a component of the bile acids that help you digest fats, it's a major piece of the outer layer of every one of your cells, and it's also an important part of vitamin D and certain hormones like estrogen and testosterone.

There are two major types of cholesterol: LDL and HDL. LDL cholesterol is categorized as "bad" cholesterol, while HDL is classified as "good" cholesterol. Many cholesterol tests also measure triglycerides. While not technically cholesterol, triglycerides are another type of fat in your blood that is used to store extra energy—or calories—from the food you eat. High levels of triglycerides are associated with both heart disease and insulin resistance.

When you get a standard cholesterol test (a lipid profile), your doctor looks at all the numbers: your total cholesterol, LDL cholesterol, and HDL cholesterol. If the values for total cholesterol and/or LDL cholesterol are elevated, it's considered a risk factor for developing heart disease.

The cholesterol you eat has a minimal impact on the amount of cholesterol in your blood. This is because your body doesn't absorb dietary cholesterol well. Most of the cholesterol you get from your diet travels right through your digestive system and never makes it into your blood. Your body is designed to have a certain amount of cholesterol, so if you're limiting the cholesterol in your diet, your liver will ramp up its production to compensate.

Fast Away Bad Cholesterol

Intermittent fasting can reduce total cholesterol levels by as much as 20 percent, but what's even more impressive than that is the effect intermittent fasting has on individual lipids. Studies show that an eight-week alternate-day fast can reduce LDL cholesterol levels by approximately 25 percent. Fasting also reduces the number of the small, dense LDL particles. When the body is not making new free fatty acids (like when you are on a fasting plan), it results in a decrease of VLDL, or very low-density lipoproteins, which in turn reduces LDL.

That's not all: fasting can also decrease triglycerides by as much as 32 percent, and while it lowers both problematic cholesterol markers, fasting has no negative effect on HDL, or "good" cholesterol.

Get a Healthier Brain

Fatigue, brain fog, and an inability to concentrate are some of the most common symptoms plaguing people today, but these symptoms are not normal in a properly functioning body. High blood sugar and insulin levels, insulin resistance, and excess weight all contribute to decreased brain function. Because intermittent fasting helps balance blood sugar and insulin levels—and can help you shed excess pounds—it also leads to marked improvement in these symptoms. Intermittent fasting can also have direct effects on your brain health through several mechanisms.

According to Dr. Mark Mattson—the senior investigator and lab chief at the Laboratory of Neurosciences at the National Institute on Aging, and a neuroscience professor at Johns Hopkins University School of Medicine—intermittent fasting has been shown to increase the rate of neurogenesis (the development of new brain cells and nerve tissues in the brain). Increased rates of neurogenesis are linked with boosts in mood, memory, focus, and overall brain function.

Intermittent fasting also increases the production of brain-derived neurotrophic factor (BDNF), a protein that helps control your brain and general health. When your brain is challenged—by anything from intense exercise or mental stimulation to calorie restriction—the body increases its production of BDNF. A higher level of BDNF strengthens the connection between existing neurons and increases the brain's production of new neurons. Furthermore, high levels of BDNF are associated with lower levels of depression and a boost in mood and motivation.

The increase in human growth hormone caused by intermittent fasting has also been shown to improve cognition, protect the brain from damage, and increase the production of new brain cells.

What Is Starvation Mode?

Starvation mode is one of the most common concerns of people who are new to intermittent fasting. To be clear, starvation mode (adaptive thermogenesis) is a real thing; however, how it works is often misunderstood.

When you eat food, your body either uses it for any immediate energy needs or stores it in fat tissue for later use. If a greater number of calories enter the fat tissue than the number of calories that leave it, you gain fat. If the opposite happens, you lose fat. This is the basis of the "calories in, calories out" theory (although the science is becoming more and more clear that not all calories are created equally). When you're trying to lose weight, you typically restrict calories in some way. This prompts an imbalance between calories in and calories out that will likely allow you to lose weight. You see this as a good thing, but your body sees it as a bad thing.

Your body's main concern is survival, and when you start to burn off extra calories and lose fat in the process, your body sees it as a threat—the beginning of an impending starvation. As a result, in an effort to save itself, your body starts to conserve calories and doesn't burn them off as effectively, so over time—and after significant weight loss—your calorie needs go down. This is adaptive thermogenesis.

The Muscle Loss Myth

It's a common belief that if you miss a meal, your body will immediately start turning to your muscles as an energy source, but thanks to human evolution it doesn't work like that.

In order for the body to achieve its main goal of survival, it has to obtain energy. Its preferred source is glucose, which comes mainly from carbohydrates. If glucose is not available, the body will then turn to body fat, which is essentially stored energy. Remember: when you eat an excess of calories, your body converts them to triglycerides and stores those triglycerides in your fat cells. The body instinctively knows to use muscle as an energy source only when glucose and body fat are too low to sustain life. This happens only when body fat dips below 4 percent, which is extremely low. To put it into perspective, male athletes typically have a body fat percentage of 6–13 percent, while female athletes have around 14–20 percent. Your body will preserve muscle mass until body fat becomes so low that it has no choice but to use protein for fuel. Most people never reach this point.

It's true that when you restrict calories without incorporating any form of resistance training, there's a possibility that you'll lose some muscle mass, but fasting doesn't increase the amount of muscle mass that you lose. In fact, research shows that people who incorporate fasting into their weight loss plan experience less of a reduction in lean muscle mass than those who don't intermittently fast.

The Risks of Low Blood Sugar

One of the most common concerns when it comes to intermittent fasting centers around blood sugar. At some point in your life, you've probably experienced the symptoms of low blood sugar—hunger, irritability, weakness, sweaty palms, or anxiety—when you've gone too long without eating. While it's true that low blood sugar can be unpleasant, it's not the fact that you've gone without eating that causes your blood sugar to dip too low: it's what you ate during your previous meal.

When you eat a meal that's loaded with carbohydrates, it sends a rush of glucose into your bloodstream. Your body responds to the glucose rush by releasing insulin to carry it into the cells so you can use it as energy. The higher your glucose spikes, the more insulin that's sent out; the more insulin that's sent out, the more your blood sugar ultimately drops over time. When you combine fasting with a healthy, moderate- to low-carbohydrate diet, your body is extremely efficient in managing blood glucose levels on its own, so you don't experience those dramatic spikes and dips in your blood sugar even when you go for an extended period of time without eating.

If you have problems with blood sugar control or if you're diabetic, the glucose and insulin response doesn't work as well, so make sure to speak with your healthcare provider before starting any type of fast to determine if it's right for you.

Is Fasting Bad for Women?

Because women's bodies were physiologically designed to carry babies, they're more sensitive to potential starvation than men. If a woman's body senses any impending starvation, it will respond by increasing the hormones leptin and ghrelin, which work together to control hunger. This hormonal response is the female body's way of protecting a developing fetus, even if a woman is not currently pregnant.

Although it's possible to ignore the hunger signals from ghrelin and leptin, it becomes increasingly difficult, especially as the body revolts and starts to produce more of these hormones. If a woman gives in to the hunger in an unhealthy way—by overeating or consuming unhealthy foods—this can cause a cascade of other hormonal issues involving insulin.

This process can also shut down the reproductive system. If your body thinks it doesn't have enough food to survive, it might shut down the ability to conceive to protect a potential pregnancy. This is why fasting is not recommended during pregnancy or for women who are trying to become pregnant.

The hypothalamic-pituitary-gonadal (HPG) axis controls the endocrine glands involved in ovulation. The first part of the ovulation process is the release of gonadotropin-releasing hormone (GnRH) from the hypothalamus. The release of GnRH then triggers the pituitary gland to release both follicle-stimulating hormone (FSH) and luteinizing hormone (LH). In women, the release of FSH and LH trigger the ovaries and the production of estrogen and progesterone. The increase in estrogen and progesterone is what causes the release of a mature egg (ovulation). This hormonal cascade usually happens in a regular cycle. However, GnRH is extremely sensitive and can be thrown off by fasting.

Crescendo Fasting

This doesn't mean that intermittent fasting isn't right for you if you're a woman; it just means that you should ease into it a little more carefully. If you're a woman who's fasting for the first time, trying to figure out if it's right for you, you may want to start with crescendo fasting.

With crescendo fasting, you fast only for twelve to sixteen hours a few days per week, rather than every day. These fast days should be nonconsecutive (Tuesday, Thursday, and Saturday, for example). On fasting days, you should engage only in light exercise, like yoga or walking. Strenuous exercise, like strength training, should be reserved for nonfasting days, when you're eating normally. It's also important to drink plenty of water—the typical recommendation is the equivalent of half of your body weight in ounces, so if you weigh 140 pounds, you should drink a minimum of 70 ounces of water each day. Of course, the amount of water you need depends on a variety of factors, including your age, weight, activity level, and the amount of coffee you drink, but you should use this equation as a baseline.

If you feel good after crescendo fasting for a couple of weeks, you can add in another day of fasting and see how your body reacts. If you still feel good, you can add in more days until you reach your fasting goals. The main point of crescendo fasting is to ease in slowly and avoid shocking the body too much at once.

Eat Mindfully

A meal should be something that you savor, not something that you rush through at your desk while working or in your car between errands. Part of optimal health is eating slowly and mindfully so that you can enjoy every bite—and you can pay attention to signals that tell you when you've had enough. Since you'll be eating fewer meals when you're intermittent fasting, it's even more of a reason to slow down and enjoy the process.

Treat your meals like they're an important part of your day and not just an afterthought. When it's time to eat, stop everything else and sit down for a proper meal. Prepare your body for digestion by taking a deep breath and transitioning into a relaxed state.

Should I Clean My Plate?

Forget about cleaning your plate. From a young age, you're taught to clear everything off of your plate. You may have been told not to waste food or that there are starving children in other parts of the world who would love a hot meal. While the sentiment behind those statements is meant to be positive, they can backfire in the long term. You carry those ideas into adulthood and may have a tendency to eat every bite of food on your plate, even if you're full halfway through the meal. This isn't to say you should waste food, but instead of overstuffing yourself in the interest of clearing your plate, serve yourself a smaller portion to begin with, or save what you can't eat for your next meal. Listen to your body and the signals that tell you you're full—and honor those signals.

Smaller Plates Are Better

It may be a trick of the mind, but smaller plates can help with portion control. When you're holding a plate, you tend to fill it. That means that when you have a large plate, you'll typically serve yourself more food than if you had a smaller plate. Instead of a dinner plate, opt for a salad or appetizer plate. You can go always go back for seconds if you're still hungry, but give yourself some time to allow your food to settle. Often it's a good practice to let five to ten minutes pass between the time you finish your food and the time you go back for a second helping. That gives your body a chance to decide if you're really hungry.

Take Your Time

Today's world is "go, go, go." People tend to rush through their entire days—and eating is no different. Next time you sit down for a meal, take a breath and slow down. Put your utensils down between bites and chew slowly instead of rushing to get in and swallow each bite as quickly as you can.

Pay attention to what you're eating. When was the last time you paid attention to the texture of the food you were eating? The crunch of almonds, the tanginess of your salad dressing, and the coolness of a bite of avocado often go unnoticed when you're rushing through your meal to get to the next moment. Make it a point to pay attention, not just to the flavor of your food but to the whole experience. Eating a meal is supposed to be pleasurable. Take it all in.

Fasting and Binges

There's a popular belief that if you go too long without eating, you'll end up binging on unhealthy foods once you do eat, ultimately gaining weight. It's not so black and white: there are many factors to consider.

Studies on alternate-day fasting show that people who fast tend to take in more calories on the day after a twenty-four-hour fast; however, the increase is under 500 calories. So if you factor the calories missed during fasting into the minimal increase in intake the next day, it still comes out to a calorie deficit.

The desire to binge is often also caused by the dramatic dip in blood sugar that occurs after a carbohydrate-rich meal or due to a carbohydrate addiction. Once your blood sugar levels off after a period of time of intermittent fasting, you'll notice that hunger stabilizes and you have less of a desire to eat in excess.

For those who have struggled with bulimia or binge-eating disorder, it's possible that fasting can lead to binges or bulimic behavior. Make sure to speak with your healthcare provider before starting intermittent fasting if you have a history of disordered eating.

Choosing the Right Diet

Although the term *diet* is commonly associated with some type of food restriction, keep in mind that the main definition of *diet* is "the type of food a person habitually eats," and that's how you should interpret the term here. There's no specific diet that you must follow when intermittent fasting, but of course you'll reap the most benefits if you choose a diet full of nutrient-rich, unprocessed foods. There are some diets that are popular complements to intermittent fasting, but don't get caught up in dogma. You don't have to follow a diet plan exactly as written. For example, if you decide to follow a Paleo template but discover that your body does well with brown rice, you can add it in. You don't have to omit a food for good just because it doesn't fall under a dietary title. Use intuitive eating to figure out your best approach.

5

Ingredients for a Healthy Fasting Diet

The intermittent fasting lifestyle isn't just about not eating; it's also about being more aware of what foods you *do* eat. Just as there are various methods of fasting, there are different diets you can follow, including Paleo, low-carb, and pegan. You need to find the one that works for you and accomplishes what you want. In addition, you need to make good choices when food shopping, finding foods and drinks that promote maximum health.

Maintain a Ratio of Carbs, Protein, and Fats

Most of the major diets put an emphasis on macronutrients (carbohydrates, proteins, and fats). There are low-carbohydrate, high-fat diets and low-fat, high-carbohydrate diets. There is also IIFYM, "if it fits your macros," which is based on the principle that you can eat whatever you want as long as you maintain the ratio of carbohydrates, proteins, and fats that is right for your body. Although some of these diets do focus on food quality, many of them are missing a major piece of the health puzzle: micronutrients.

Carbohydrates, proteins, and fats are macronutrients; vitamins and minerals are micronutrients. However, just because the body needs micronutrients in smaller amounts, it doesn't mean they're less important. In fact, the importance of getting adequate amounts of micronutrients cannot be overstated.

The Importance of Micronutrients

Thirteen vitamins and sixteen minerals (called micronutrients) are needed in adequate amounts each day. These vitamins and minerals help keep all your bodily functions working in the right way. Some affect your blood, others help you metabolize carbs, proteins, and fats. Of course, this only touches the surface. These and other vitamins and minerals play many other roles in your body.

If your intake of vitamins and minerals falls short, over time you'll develop a deficiency. Although it might not seem like a big issue, even a small deficiency in one micronutrient can cause major health problems. Low levels of vitamin D have been associated with depression (especially seasonal affective disorder, which occurs in the winter months) and irritable bowel syndrome. Magnesium deficiency can cause irregular heartbeat, muscle twitching and cramps, high blood pressure, fatigue, depression, and apathy (lack of emotion). Deficiencies in vitamin B_{12} can present psychological conditions, such as dementia, paranoia, and major depression.

The Ketogenic Diet

The ketogenic diet is one of the most popular diet companions to intermittent fasting. People who love intermittent fasting tend to lean toward this diet because the two approaches complement each other nicely: when used in combination, they'll quickly kick you into a chronic state of ketosis (a physiological state in which your body burns fat for energy instead of carbohydrates).

When following a ketogenic diet, most of your calories will come from fat, and your carbohydrate intake will be severely restricted. Unlike other diets, a ketogenic diet requires you to keep track of exactly how much fat, carbohydrates, and protein you're eating.

A typical ketogenic diet has a macronutrient breakdown as follows:

- 60–75 percent of calories from fat
- 15–30 percent of calories from protein
- 5–10 percent of calories from carbohydrates

The Paleo Diet

The Paleo diet is another popular companion to intermittent fasting because, like fasting, it's designed from the eating habits of your ancestors. The basic concept of a Paleo diet is to consume only foods that were available to hunters and gatherers during the Paleolithic era. Of course, this definition is open to interpretation because your Paleolithic ancestors wouldn't have access to things like jars of almond butter, but you get the idea.

When following a Paleo diet, you can eat:

- Eggs
- Fish
- Fruits
- Healthy fats (avocado oil, coconut oil, olive oil, ghee)
- Meat
- Natural sweeteners (raw honey, maple syrup, coconut sugar)
- Nuts and seeds
- Poultry

On the other hand, you'll need to avoid:

- Alcohol
- Dairy (milk, cheese, ice cream, butter)
- Grains (wheat, oats, barley, rye, quinoa, couscous, amaranth, millet, corn)
- Legumes (soy, peanuts, chickpeas, beans)
- Refined and artificial sweeteners (white sugar, high-fructose corn syrup, sucralose, aspartame)

The Pegan Diet

The pegan diet is a fairly new concept that was developed by Dr. Mark Hyman, the director of the Cleveland Clinic Center for Functional Medicine. The pegan diet combines the basic principles of the Paleo diet and a vegan diet, which seems counterintuitive since at first glance the diets appear to be on completely opposite ends of the spectrum; however, their basic principles are actually very similar.

Both the Paleo diet and a vegan diet emphasize choosing whole, unprocessed foods that are responsibly sourced from the land. The major differences are that the Paleo diet focuses on ethically sourced meats, vegetables, healthy fats, and some fruits, and eliminates all grains and legumes; a vegan diet eliminates all animal products and emphasizes grains, legumes, vegetables, and all plant-based foods. The goal of the pegan diet is to combine the best things from the two diets.

What You Can Eat on the Pegan Diet

When following the pegan diet, plant-based foods will make up about 75 percent of your daily intake. You'll want to eat mostly vegetables; some fruits; some gluten-free grains, like quinoa, brown rice, and gluten-free oats; and some legumes, like lentils. The other 25 percent of your food intake should be in the form of high-quality animal proteins (grass-fed beef, pasture-raised chicken, and eggs) and healthy fats, like coconut, olives, and avocados (and their respective oils: coconut oil, olive oil, and avocado oil). Dr. Hyman recommends treating meat more like a condiment than the main course. Instead of a typical 4- to 6-ounce serving, stick to 2–3 ounces of meat per meal.

While following the pegan diet, you'll avoid gluten, dairy, and some vegetable oils (canola, sunflower, corn, and soybean). Sugar—even natural types like honey and maple syrup—should be eaten only as an occasional treat. Although natural sugars do provide some health benefits, overdoing them can negatively affect blood sugar levels—something you're ultimately trying to avoid when intermittent fasting.

The Low-FODMAP Diet

FODMAPs (fermentable oligosaccharides, disaccharides, monosaccharides, and polyols), are short-chain carbohydrates that can cause digestive distress in those who have digestive sensitivities. A low-FODMAP diet is typically recommended for someone who is experiencing chronic digestive trouble or unexplained irritable bowel syndrome. When following a low-FODMAP diet, you'll avoid certain categories of carbohydrates, which include:

- **Oligosaccharides:** wheat, rye, legumes, garlic, onions, leeks, asparagus, jicama, fennel, beetroot, and Brussels sprouts
- **Disaccharides:** white sugar, milk, yogurt, and soft cheeses like cream cheese and cottage cheese
- **Monosaccharides:** peaches, plums, pears, nectarines, mangoes, watermelon, apples, and honey
- **Polyols:** blackberries, avocados, sweet potatoes, cauliflower, snow peas, and mushrooms

When following a low-FODMAP diet, you'll completely eliminate all high-FODMAP foods for about one month. After this initial elimination period, you can reintroduce one high-FODMAP food at a time to see how your body reacts. If you don't experience any digestive upset, it's likely your body can handle that food. If you do experience digestive upset, it's likely that you're sensitive to that food and you'd do well to avoid it as much as possible.

The Low-Carb Diet

A low-carb diet is similar to a ketogenic diet in that you restrict the amount of carbohydrates you take in each day. However, a traditional low-carb diet is not as high in fat and allows a more moderate intake of protein than a ketogenic diet does. Many low-carb diets suggest an initial period of very low-carbohydrate intake—around two weeks— where you remove almost all carbohydrate-containing foods, except low-carb vegetables. During this initial period, you'll lose a significant amount of water weight. After these two weeks, you'll move on to a more sustainable program in which you can include healthy sources of carbohydrates, such as other vegetables, some fruits, and gluten-free whole grains. The major goal of a standard low-carbohydrate diet is to lower blood sugar and insulin levels and promote weight loss.

Wheat

Wheat has been a part of agriculture for over nine thousand years and is one of the largest crops in the world. It's considered an integral part of many nations' food supply because it can be stored in kernel form for years and can be processed to make a wide variety of foods, including flour, breads, noodles, and cereals. The problem with wheat is not in the grain itself but what modern agriculture has done to it.

The wheat of today is not only lower in many nutrients that were in wheat of the past, but the structure of the plant itself has been changed due to modern milling. The goal of modern processes is to create a crop that can survive should disaster strike, so major food corporations have made it resistant to drought, adverse weather, pests, and chemicals. As a result of this, your body doesn't recognize wheat the way that it used to. Instead of providing nourishment, wheat has become inflammatory and addictive.

Grains

It seems that nutrition experts—and the general population—are divided down the middle when it comes to whether grains are good or bad for you. One side of the debate recommends avoiding grains, while the other side says that whole grains are a necessity due to their fiber and vitamin B content. The anti-grains side says that there are three major problems with grains: lectins, phytates, and gluten.

Lectins—proteins that bind to cell membranes—are found in both grains and legumes. They are small and hard to digest because they're resistant to both heat and digestive enzymes. Because of this, they tend to accumulate in your body and travel into your blood in their whole form. When proteins enter your blood whole, your immune system develops antibodies, which means that it recognizes the protein as a foreign invader and builds up an attack system against it. Over time this can result in leaky gut and increased sensitivity to lectins.

Phytates are compounds found mainly in grains and legumes, and in lesser amounts in nuts and seeds. Phytates are not inherently bad for you, but they're often described as anti-nutrients because they bind to minerals like iron, zinc, and calcium, preventing their absorption. This can set you up for mineral deficiencies. It's important to note here that phytates don't impair your ability to absorb nutrients over the long term; they only block absorption during that meal.

Going Gluten-Free

Of course, when it comes to grains, gluten is the most controversial. While celiac disease—an inability to properly digest gluten—is widely accepted, many people don't believe in non-celiac gluten sensitivity. But research shows that gluten can damage the intestinal lining (and cause celiac disease symptoms) even in people who don't have the disease.

Gluten-free grains include brown rice, wild rice, quinoa, buckwheat, millet, teff, and amaranth. Oats are technically gluten-free as well, but because of the way they're manufactured, they're almost always contaminated by gluten. If you want to include oats in your diet, choose brands that are specifically labeled as gluten-free.

Make Your Grains Healthier

Soak your grains before consumption. Soaking grains can help break down the phytates and neutralize the lectins, so the grains are easier to digest and you are able to absorb all of the minerals in them. To soak the grains, place them in a bowl and cover completely with warm, filtered water. For every cup of water you add to the bowl, you must also add a tablespoon of an acidic medium, such as lemon juice or apple cider vinegar. For example, if you need 3 cups of water to cover your grains, add 3 tablespoons of lemon juice to the water, then cover the bowl with a breathable medium, like a clean kitchen towel. Next, let the grains sit for twelve hours. After the grains have soaked for an adequate amount of time, rinse them off with cold water and proceed with your recipe as usual.

Another option is to sprout your grains or to use grains that have already been sprouted. Food manufacturers have caught onto the health benefits of sprouting your grains, and many companies now offer grains that are already sprouted, which can save you time and effort. If you can't find already sprouted grains in your local grocery store, you can look online or sprout them yourself.

Sprout Your Grains

Sprouting takes considerably longer than soaking grains because you have to wait for the grain to actually crack open and form a sprout. To sprout your own grains, follow the process for soaking and then transfer the soaked and drained grains to a glass jar—a Mason jar works well. Cover the jar with a cheesecloth and allow the grains to sit in the moist jar at room temperature for one to five days. You'll know when they're ready because the grains will crack open and a green sprout will be visible. You can store sprouted grains in the refrigerator for up to one week.

Dairy

Dairy is another controversial product in the nutrition world. You probably grew up hearing about how great milk is for your bones. The truth is that milk is not as good for your bones as you may think. In fact, the countries with the lowest milk consumption have the lowest rates of fractures and osteoporosis, a condition in which the bones become brittle and are more prone to breaks and fractures. In addition, many people have trouble digesting the proteins and sugars found in milk. This is because as you age, your body's production of lactase—the enzyme that you need to digest milk properly—naturally decreases.

However, this doesn't mean that you can't consume any dairy, but there are some options that are better than others. If you are going to include dairy in your diet, choose dairy that comes from grass-fed cows. You can usually find grass-fed milk, butter, and cheese at local stores. Grass-fed dairy has a higher content of omega-3s, unlike conventional dairy, which has more omega-6s. Omega-6s aren't inherently bad, but when you eat too many (which many Americans do), it can lead to chronic inflammation. Cultured grass-fed dairy products, like yogurt and kefir, are also good choices; however, make sure they are full-fat and plain. Flavored yogurts and kefirs are often loaded with sugar.

Go with Goats

If you want to avoid cow's milk completely, goat's milk products are a great option. Modern cow's milk contains high amounts of a protein called *A1 beta-casein*, which can be very inflammatory and cause issues like eczema and acne. On the other hand, goat's milk contains a protein called *A2 beta-casein*, which is not inflammatory. Studies show that people who consume milk with A2 beta-casein experienced reduced inflammation and no negative digestive symptoms.

Goat's milk is also more environmentally responsible than cow's milk since goats consume less grass and take up less space than cows. The land required to support two cows can support six goats.

Meat and Poultry

Meat is another controversial product that has been vilified over the years due to its saturated-fat content. When low-fat diets became really popular, red meat was a major no-no; but since then, science has shown that saturated fat doesn't have as great an impact on heart disease as previously thought. In fact, the right types of saturated fat can protect against heart disease.

The old school of thought was that saturated fat raised cholesterol, which increased the risk of heart disease; but research now shows that while saturated fats can raise the amount of LDL in your blood, it creates the large, fluffy LDL particles that don't stick to the artery walls (compared to the small, dense LDL particles that do get stuck on the artery walls and can cause blockages, increasing your heart disease risk). Saturated fat also raises HDL levels, which is what protects against heart disease.

Meat is also one of the top sources of vitamin B_{12}. In fact, you can only get vitamin B_{12} from animal products (though it is added to some foods, including some fortified cereals). Meat also contains the other B vitamins, vitamin D, vitamin E, amino acids, antioxidants, and several minerals.

Choose Grass-Fed Meat

Just as with dairy, it's important to choose high-quality, grass-fed meats. Conventional meat comes from cows that are fed GMO (genetically modified organism) crops, grains, and even sugar. This fattens the cows up quicker so they produce more, but it affects the nutritional content of their meat. Grass-fed meat contains up to five times more omega-3 fatty acids than conventional meat, and significantly fewer omega-6s.

Grass-fed meat also contains a fat called conjugated linoleic acid, or CLA. CLA acts as an antioxidant and has been shown to reduce the risk of heart disease, stop the growth of cancerous tumors, prevent atherosclerosis, decrease triglycerides, and reduce the risk of developing type 2 diabetes. All animal foods contain some amount of CLA, but grass-fed meat and dairy contain up to 500 percent more than dairy and meat that comes from grain-fed cows.

Poultry

As with meat, not all poultry is the same. There is poultry that comes from conventional farms, and then there is poultry that's raised organically and allowed to roam freely, eating a natural diet. Often you'll see labels on poultry and eggs that boast that the birds were "fed a vegetarian diet," but chickens and turkeys are not vegetarians. They like to scavenge for bugs, ticks, and worms, and that is what makes their meat so nutritious. Poultry that has been allowed to consume a natural diet is higher in omega-3s, vitamins, and minerals.

When choosing poultry, it's best to choose a combination of organic and pasture-raised. If this is unavailable at your local grocery store or your budget doesn't allow for it, talk to your local farmers. Often you may find high-quality meats at your local farms that aren't labeled as pasture-raised or organic (because these are government-moderated terms, and many small farms can't afford to pay for the certification process required to carry these labels), but by definition are both of these things.

Eggs

There is a lot of fear surrounding cholesterol, so people often separate their eggs, throwing away the yolk and eating only the egg white. While the white of the egg contains protein, most of the nutrients, like vitamins A, D, E, and K; B vitamins; omega-3 fats; calcium; and phosphorus, are found in its yolk. Don't be scared to eat the whole egg, but do choose the types of eggs you consume wisely.

Many of the labels and nutritional claims on eggs are just marketing tactics. For example, the terms *natural* and *farm fresh* usually mean nothing. Other terms, like *cage-free*, sound good, but they can be misleading. When you hear the term *cage-free*, you may picture birds roaming around outside in the sunlight, but cage-free just means that the birds were not in cages. They could still have been in an overcrowded warehouse without much room to move. The best type of eggs you can get are organic and pasture-raised. Again, talking to your local egg farmers is a great way to find high-quality eggs that are usually fresher and less expensive than the eggs you'll find in a grocery store.

Seafood

Seafood is loaded with protein and beneficial vitamins and minerals, but the most notable health benefits tied to seafood come from two specific omega-3 fatty acids: eicosapentaenoic acid (EPA) and docosahexaenoic acid (DHA). Regular consumption of EPA and DHA has been shown to reduce the risk of heart disease, cancer, type 2 diabetes, and autoimmune diseases.

When choosing fish, it's best to consume smaller species of fish. Larger fish that are higher on the food chain tend to accumulate more mercury and other heavy metals and toxins in their flesh.

The fish and shellfish that are highest in omega-3s include:

- Herring
- Mackerel
- Mussels
- Oysters
- Salmon
- Sardines
- Trout

Wild Beats Farm-Raised

In addition to choosing smaller fish that are high in omega-3 fatty acids, it's also best to choose fish that have been wild caught rather than farm-raised. As with animals that are raised for conventional meat, farmed fish are fed a diet that is not natural to them. This may include corn and grains. As a result of their unnatural diet, farm-raised fish become high in omega-6 fatty acids and lower in omega-3 fatty acids. In fact, according to one analysis published in the *Journal of the American Dietetic Association*, omega-3 fatty acids couldn't even be detected in some farm-raised fish found in grocery stores. In addition to the altered levels of fatty acids, farm-raised fish accumulate higher levels of toxins and contaminants in their flesh.

Fruits and Vegetables

You know that fruits and vegetables are good for you. Of course, some fruit contains more natural sugar than others, but when this sugar is combined with the fiber in the fruit, it's not a problem for most people. Problems arise from drinking too much fruit juice, which contains all of the sugar without any of the fiber, so when eating fruit, make sure to eat it whole and ideally with the skin on (which contains fiber).

There's also research that shows that organic produce not only contains fewer pesticides and herbicides than conventional produce, but that it is also richer in some vitamins and minerals.

The Dirty Dozen and the Clean Fifteen

If your budget doesn't allow for a lot of organic choices, you can prioritize which fruits and vegetables to purchase organic by using the Environmental Working Group's Dirty Dozen list. The Dirty Dozen list outlines which fruits and vegetables typically have the most contamination. These are the produce items that you should prioritize buying organic. The Dirty Dozen (in descending order) are:

- Strawberries
- Spinach
- Nectarines
- Apples
- Grapes
- Peaches
- Cherries
- Pears
- Tomatoes
- Celery
- Potatoes
- Sweet bell peppers

In addition to the Dirty Dozen list, the Environmental Working Group also supplies a list of the produce that tends to contain the lowest amount of pesticides and contaminants. These fruits and vegetables are the ones that you don't have to prioritize buying organic. This list is called the Clean Fifteen (beginning with the cleanest):

- Avocados
- Sweet corn
- Pineapples
- Cabbages
- Onions
- Frozen sweet peas
- Papayas
- Asparagus
- Mangoes
- Eggplants
- Honeydew melons
- Kiwis
- Cantaloupes
- Cauliflower
- Broccoli

Fats and Oils

Fat is nothing to fear. In fact, including healthy fats in your diet can provide valuable vitamins and minerals and help keep you full longer. The key is to choose fats that are good for you. Natural, healthy fats are vital components of a balanced diet.

Margarine contains trans fats in the form of hydrogenated oils. Trans fats were created to give foods a longer shelf life, but they have a detrimental effect on cholesterol levels. Unlike saturated fats, which increase the large, fluffy LDL particles that don't stick to the artery walls, trans fats increase the small, dense LDL particles that get stuck on the artery walls and can cause blockages that increase your risk for heart disease.

Refined oils like soybean oil, which is a common ingredient in many prepackaged foods, are high in omega-6 fatty acids. As you've already learned, eating too many omega-6 fatty acids can contribute to chronic inflammation, which is connected to a number of diseases and health issues.

The best fats to consume include:

- Avocado oil
- Coconut oil
- Grass-fed ghee
- Hemp oil
- Olive oil
- Sesame oil
- Unsalted grass-fed butter
- Walnut oil

Sugar

Most of the health problems that are often blamed on fat are really due to sugar. Sugar doesn't have any health benefits, yet the average American consumes approximately 66 pounds of sugar per year. Even more concerning than having no nutritional value is the fact that sugar contributes to chronic inflammation, increases your risk of heart disease, destabilizes blood sugar levels, and feeds cancer cells. Eating too much sugar can also make it easy for you to gain weight.

Manufacturers have tried to solve the problem of sugar by introducing artificial sweeteners to the market, but studies show that people who consume artificial sweeteners have a greater risk of diabetes, metabolic syndrome, and heart disease. Artificial sweeteners can also throw off the balance of bacteria in your gut, causing both digestive and systemic issues. Artificial sweeteners have even been linked to cancer and chronic migraines. In addition to that, when you give your body the sweet taste without any calories, it can lead to sugar cravings that are even more intense.

Best Choices for Sweeteners

No matter what form it's in, sugar should be limited as much as possible. However, there are certain sweeteners that are better for you than others. The best choices include:

- Coconut sugar
- Date sugar
- Erythritol (sparingly)
- Molasses
- Monk fruit
- Palm sugar
- Pure maple syrup
- Raw honey
- Stevia (sparingly)

Although stevia is a plant and is marketed as natural, many packaged forms are highly processed by the time they're available to you. In addition to that, some stevia products also contain added ingredients, like "natural flavors," that are unfavorable. The term *natural flavors* is not closely regulated by the FDA, and companies are free to use this description even for chemical additives that mimic natural flavors. If you choose to use stevia, do so sparingly and make sure you're choosing one that's pure and organic.

6

50+ Intermittent Fasting Recipes

Here are more than fifty recipes that will work well with your new intermittent fasting lifestyle. They're a mixture of traditional and vegetarian, including such favorites as South of the Border Scrambler, Bacon and Vegetable Omelet, and Lemon Thyme Chicken. From breakfasts to dinner with soups, salads, and snacks in between, every meal is covered. And of course, there's always room for desserts like Peanut Butter Cookies and Peach Tart.

Breakfast Casserole

You can prepare this delicious casserole a day or two in advance so you have a quick breakfast ready to go that doesn't require any extra prep.

Serves 4

- 1 pound 85 percent lean ground beef
- 1 small yellow onion, peeled and diced
- 1 teaspoon freshly ground black pepper
- 1 teaspoon garlic powder
- 1 teaspoon red pepper flakes
- 12 large eggs
- 1 cup unsweetened full-fat coconut milk
- 1 tablespoon coconut oil
- 1 small butternut squash, peeled, seeded, and sliced

1. In a large skillet over medium heat, start cooking ground beef. Add onion and spices, cooking 10 minutes until onions are soft.
2. In a large bowl, whisk together eggs and milk.
3. Grease the inside of a 4- to 6-quart slow cooker with coconut oil. Add in squash, beef mixture, and egg mixture. Stir and make sure that beef mixture is completely covered by egg mixture. Cook on low heat 10 hours.
4. Scoop out, slice, and serve warm.

PER SERVING

Calories: 581 | Fat: 37.4g | Protein: 41.3g | Sodium: 288mg | Fiber: 1.6g | Carbohydrates: 11.4g | Net Carbohydrates: 9.8g | Sugar: 2.5g

Autumn Breakfast Chia Bowl

This Autumn Breakfast Chia Bowl contains cranberry and cinnamon flavors reminiscent of the fall, but it can be enjoyed any time of the year.

Serves 2

3 cups cold water
¼ teaspoon salt
1 cup gluten-free steel-cut oats
½ cup unsweetened almond milk
3 tablespoons chia seeds

1 tablespoon halved macadamia nuts
1 tablespoon sliced almonds
½ teaspoon ground cinnamon
1 tablespoon no-sugar-added dried cranberries

1. In a medium saucepan, bring water and salt to a boil on high heat, then add oats. Reduce heat to medium-low, add milk, and stir.
2. Add chia seeds, macadamia nuts, almonds, cinnamon, and cranberries to pan and stir.
3. Cover and cook on medium-low heat 20 minutes, stirring occasionally until chia seeds become soft and gel-like. Serve immediately.

PER SERVING

Calories: 471 | Fat: 15.6g | Protein: 17.8g | Sodium: 352mg | Fiber: 16.8g | Carbohydrates: 67.2g | Net Carbohydrates: 50.4g | Sugar: 0.6g

Turkey, Egg White, and Hash Brown Bake

When you have a craving for a hearty, but still healthy, breakfast, make this satisfying dish. Quick and easy to whip up, this bake is perfect for your first meal—or any meal—of the day.

Serves 16

1 tablespoon olive oil

1 pound 85 percent lean ground turkey

1 pound russet potatoes, peeled and shredded

12 large eggs

1½ teaspoons salt

1½ teaspoons freshly ground black pepper

½ teaspoon ground cayenne pepper

1. Preheat oven to 375°F.
2. Grease a 9" × 13" glass casserole dish with cooking spray.
3. Heat oil in a medium skillet over medium heat 1 minute. Add ground turkey and cook until no longer pink, about 6 minutes.
4. Transfer cooked turkey to a large bowl and combine with remaining ingredients. Mix well.
5. Pour mixture into prepared baking dish. Bake 40 minutes until top is set and an inserted toothpick comes out clean.
6. Allow to cool 5 minutes, then cut into 16 pieces and serve.

PER SERVING

Calories: 137 | Fat: 7.4g | Protein: 10.7g | Sodium: 344mg | Fiber: 0.5g | Carbohydrates: 5.1g | Net Carbohydrates: 4.6g | Sugar: 0.4g

Cran-Orange Oatmeal

If your standard oatmeal recipe feels a bit bland, try this revamped version! Tart cranberries and fresh orange add extra vitamins and minerals—and a zesty flavor that kicks things up a notch.

Serves 2

1 cup freshly squeezed orange juice
½ cup water
1 cup fresh cranberries
2 cups gluten-free rolled oats

1 tablespoon maple syrup
1 tablespoon freshly grated orange zest

1. Combine orange juice, water, and cranberries in a medium saucepan over medium heat. Bring to a simmer and cook for about 5 minutes.
2. Add oats and simmer, stirring constantly, until thickened, about 8 minutes. Remove from heat and stir in maple syrup.
3. Divide oatmeal into two bowls, garnish with orange zest, and serve immediately.

PER SERVING

Calories: 487 | Fat: 7.2g | Protein: 15.1g | Sodium: 3mg | Fiber: 12.9g | Carbohydrates: 90.5g | Net Carbohydrates: 77.6g | Sugar: 20.5g

South of the Border Scrambler

Short on time? This scrambled version of huevos rancheros can be made in minutes. If you want a kick, spice it up with some sliced jalapeños.

Serves 2

4 large eggs
½ teaspoon salt
¼ teaspoon freshly ground black pepper
1 teaspoon olive oil

¼ cup no-sugar-added salsa
½ large avocado, peeled, pitted, and diced
¼ cup chopped fresh cilantro

1. Whisk eggs, salt, and pepper together in a medium bowl.
2. Heat olive oil 30 seconds in a medium skillet over medium heat. Add eggs and scramble until cooked, about 4 minutes.
3. Transfer to two bowls and top each with ⅛ cup salsa, ¼ cup diced avocado, and ⅛ cup cilantro. Serve immediately.

PER SERVING
Calories: 239 | Fat: 15.6g | Protein: 13.3g | Sodium: 956mg | Fiber: 2.8g | Carbohydrates: 6.9g | Net Carbohydrates: 4.1g | Sugar: 2.5g

Simple Salsa Recipe
Here's a simple recipe for homemade salsa: combine 2 tomatoes, ½ seeded jalapeño, 2 cilantro sprigs, the juice of ½ lemon, ¼ teaspoon salt, and ⅛ teaspoon pepper. Put all ingredients in a food processor and pulse until combined.

Coconut Cacao Hazelnut Smoothie Bowl

This nutty and chocolaty bowl is delicious and loaded with healthy fats and micronutrients. Enjoy it as your first meal of the day to get a jump-start on your daily nutrient needs. For a thicker consistency, add more ice during blending.

Serves 1

1 tablespoon shredded unsweet-ened coconut

1 cup unsweetened almond milk

1 frozen ripe medium banana, peeled

2 teaspoons raw unsweetened cacao powder

1½ teaspoons pure maple syrup

⅛ teaspoon sea salt

6 ice cubes (approximately ½ cup)

5 hazelnuts, shelled and chopped

1 tablespoon shelled pumpkin seeds

1. Toast coconut in a small skillet over medium heat, stirring frequently until flakes are golden brown, about 3 minutes. Set aside.
2. Add milk, banana, cacao powder, maple syrup, salt, and ice to blender and blend until smooth, about 30 seconds.
3. Pour mixture into a serving bowl and top with hazelnuts, pumpkin seeds, and toasted coconut. Serve.

PER SERVING

Calories: 294 | Fat: 14.2g | Protein: 6.5g | Sodium: 379mg | Fiber: 6.6g | Carbohydrates: 41.1g | Net Carbohydrates: 34.5g | Sugar: 21.3g

Cacao versus Cocoa

Cacao and cocoa come from the same plant, but the major difference is in how they're processed. Cacao is minimally processed and made by cold-pressing cacao beans. Cocoa starts out as cacao but is heated at much higher temperatures than cacao, which results in a sweeter flavor. Both cacao and cocoa have health benefits, but the heat used during the processing of cocoa destroys some of the antioxidants and enzymes in it, making cacao a nutritionally superior choice.

Overnight Almond Butter Pumpkin Spice Oats

You will love digging into these hearty and delicious pumpkin oats! This dish is perfect for tiding you over during a busy day.

Serves 2

½ cup gluten-free rolled oats
¼ cup unsweetened almond milk
¼ cup pumpkin purée
½ teaspoon pumpkin pie spice
½ teaspoon alcohol-free vanilla extract

½ teaspoon ground cinnamon
1 tablespoon pure maple syrup
2 tablespoons unsalted, no-sugar-added almond butter
2 tablespoons chopped walnuts

1. In a medium bowl, combine oats and milk and stir. Add pumpkin purée, pumpkin pie spice, vanilla, cinnamon, and maple syrup. Stir.
2. Spoon half of oats mixture into each of two small canning jars. Add 1 tablespoon almond butter on top of oats in each jar. Divide remaining oats on top of almond butter. Cover with jar lids. Refrigerate overnight.
3. In the morning, top with walnuts and enjoy! Mixture can be refrigerated up to 3 days.

PER SERVING

Calories: 288 | Fat: 14.9g | Protein: 8.4g | Sodium: 25mg | Fiber: 5.9g | Carbohydrates: 30.4g | Net Carbohydrates: 24.5g | Sugar: 8.9g

Overnight Oats Have So Many Possibilities!

Overnight oats are so easy to make, and there are several different variations you can try with any of your favorite ingredients. Start with a base of oats and your favorite nondairy milk, and then add any combination of nuts, berries, spices, and a dash of a healthy sweetener (like pure maple syrup or honey). Overnight oats keep well in the refrigerator, so you can make a few at a time and keep them in jars, ready to grab on your way out the door.

Spicy Kale Scramble

This great post-workout meal provides healthy proteins and greens—with a kick!

Serves 1

1 tablespoon olive oil
1 cup chopped fresh kale
3 large eggs, beaten
2 teaspoons ground turmeric

½ teaspoon salt
¼ teaspoon freshly ground black pepper
⅛ teaspoon ground cayenne pepper

1. Heat olive oil in a medium skillet over medium heat 1 minute. Add kale and cook until wilted, about 3 minutes.
2. Add whisked eggs to skillet, then add remaining ingredients. Scramble eggs until cooked through, about 4 minutes.
3. Serve immediately.

PER SERVING

Calories: 359 | Fat: 26.5g | Protein: 20.2g | Sodium: 1,382mg | Fiber: 2.1g | Carbohydrates: 7.0g | Net Carbohydrates: 4.9g | Sugar: 1.1g

Add More Greens

This is a basic recipe that you can make even more nutritious by adding your favorite greens. Spinach, arugula, and collard greens are all great choices.

Chicken Sausage Patties

These delicious sausages pair well with sides of poached eggs and Vegetarian Hash (see recipe in this chapter). Serve with spicy chutney for an added kick.

Makes 24 patties

3 pounds ground chicken
1 medium yellow onion, peeled and finely minced
½ cup finely chopped fresh flat-leaf parsley
1 tablespoon chopped fresh sage
6 cloves garlic, peeled and minced
1 tablespoon peeled and minced fresh ginger
2 teaspoons red pepper flakes
1 teaspoon ground cloves
1 teaspoon ground white pepper
4 tablespoons olive oil

1. In a large mixing bowl, combine all ingredients except oil; mix well by hand.
2. Form mixture into 24 patties that are approximately 2" round.
3. Heat oil in a large sauté pan over medium heat until hot, about 30 seconds. Sauté patties approximately 5 minutes on each side until cooked through.
4. Serve with sides.

PER 1 PATTY

Calories: 105 | Fat: 6.4g | Protein: 10.1g | Sodium: 35mg | Fiber: 0.2g | Carbohydrates: 1.0g | Net Carbohydrates: 0.8g | Sugar: 0.2g

Artichoke and Cheese Squares

These rich vegetable squares are easy to prepare and can be made up to three days ahead of time.

Serves 8

1 (12-ounce) jar marinated artichoke hearts, drained and chopped, liquid reserved

1 small yellow onion, peeled and finely chopped

2 cloves garlic, peeled and finely minced

4 large eggs, beaten

2 tablespoons coconut flour

½ teaspoon salt

¼ teaspoon freshly ground black pepper

¼ teaspoon dried ground oregano

¼ teaspoon Tabasco

8 ounces shredded Monterey jack cheese

2 tablespoons chopped fresh flat-leaf parsley

1. Preheat oven to 325°F.
2. Heat artichoke liquid in a medium skillet over medium heat 1 minute. Sauté onion and garlic in skillet 5 minutes until onions are translucent.
3. In a mixing bowl, combine eggs, flour, salt, pepper, oregano, and Tabasco. Mix in cheese, parsley, artichokes, onion, and garlic.
4. Pour mixture into a 7" × 11" ungreased baking dish. Bake 30 minutes until egg is set. Cool 10 minutes. Cut into squares and serve warm or at room temperature.

PER SERVING
Calories: 175 | Fat: 11.2g | Protein: 12.1g | Sodium: 665mg | Fiber: 2.3g | Carbohydrates: 5.5g | Net Carbohydrates: 3.2g | Sugar: 1.0g

Zoodles with Pesto

Making "zoodles," or zucchini noodles, is not only fun but also a healthy way to enjoy pasta recipes.

Serves 3

¾ cup fresh basil leaves
2 tablespoons garlic-infused olive oil
¼ cup pine nuts
3 tablespoons olive oil, divided
½ cup freshly grated Parmesan
  cheese

¼ teaspoon sea salt, divided
¼ teaspoon freshly ground black
  pepper, divided
1 pound zucchini, peeled into long,
  narrow ribbons

1. For pesto sauce, combine basil, garlic oil, and pine nuts in a food processor and pulse until coarsely chopped, about 5 pulses. Add 2 tablespoons olive oil, cheese, ⅛ teaspoon salt, and ⅛ teaspoon pepper and process until smooth, about another 10 pulses.
2. Heat remaining olive oil in a medium sauté pan over medium heat 1 minute. Add zucchini noodles, ⅛ teaspoon salt, and ⅛ teaspoon pepper to pan and stir 5 minutes until noodles are tender. Serve with pesto sauce.

PER SERVING

Calories: 374 | Fat: 32.8g | Protein: 8.9g | Sodium: 443mg | Fiber: 2.3g | Carbohydrates: 9.1g | Net Carbohydrates: 6.8g | Sugar: 4.1g

Bacon and Vegetable Omelet

Bacon and eggs are a breakfast tradition. This omelet combines the two breakfast favorites with vegetables to help you optimize your micronutrient intake during your feeding times.

Serves 2

6 slices nitrate- and nitrite-free bacon, diced
1 medium yellow summer squash, chopped
1 cup sliced white mushrooms

1 medium zucchini, chopped
¼ cup fresh basil leaves, chopped
2 tablespoons olive oil
8 large eggs, beaten

1. In a large sauté pan over medium-high heat, cook bacon until crispy, about 5 minutes. Add vegetables and basil to pan and sauté until tender, approximately 8 minutes.
2. Heat olive oil in a second large sauté pan over medium heat, about 1 minute.
3. Add eggs to second pan and cook 3 minutes on each side.
4. Place vegetable and bacon mixture on one half of eggs and fold over other half to enclose filling. Serve.

PER SERVING

Calories: 606 | Fat: 42.5g | Protein: 40.4g | Sodium: 875mg | Fiber: 2.5g | Carbohydrates: 9.6g | Net Carbohydrates: 7.1g | Sugar: 6.1g

Salmon Omelet

This savory omelet is full of omega-3 fatty acids. It will surely become a break-fast staple.

Serves 2

2 tablespoons olive oil
¼ cup trimmed and chopped scallions
1 cup trimmed and chopped asparagus

1 tablespoon chopped fresh dill
6 ounces canned salmon
6 large eggs, beaten

1. In a large skillet, combine olive oil, scallions, asparagus, and dill. Sauté over medium-high heat until asparagus is soft, about 10 minutes, then remove mixture from skillet and set aside.
2. In same skillet on medium heat, sauté salmon until flaky, about 10 minutes, depending on thickness of salmon. Remove from skillet and set aside.
3. Let skillet cool slightly, then wipe out with a paper towel. Cook eggs on both sides over medium heat until lightly browned, about 5 minutes each side.
4. Place salmon and scallion mixture on one half of eggs and fold other half over to enclose filling. Serve.

PER SERVING
Calories: 484 | Fat: 30.2g | Protein: 42.9g | Sodium: 544mg | Fiber: 1.7g | Carbohydrates: 4.6g | Net Carbohydrates: 2.9g | Sugar: 2.1g

Vegetarian Hash

This version of an old favorite is bursting with flavor. It can be eaten as a side dish or as an entrée.

Serves 6

1½ pounds russet potatoes, peeled and large-diced

1 medium poblano (or other mild chili pepper), halved and seeded

2 medium red bell peppers, stemmed halved, seeded, and thickly sliced

1 medium red onion, peeled and thickly sliced

½ teaspoon olive oil

1 tablespoon chili powder

¼ teaspoon freshly cracked black peppercorns

¼ bunch fresh cilantro, chopped, leaves only

¼ teaspoon salt

1. Preheat oven to 400°F.
2. In a medium bowl, toss potatoes, peppers, and onions in oil, then drain on a rack. Place vegetables on an ungreased baking sheet and season with chili powder and peppercorns; roast until fork-tender, about 30 minutes.
3. Large-dice peppers and onions. Add cilantro. Season with salt and serve.

PER SERVING
Calories: 119 | Fat: 0.9g | Protein: 2.9g | Sodium: 143mg | Fiber: 3.7g | Carbohydrates: 26.2g | Net Carbohydrates: 22.5g | Sugar: 4.1g

Smoky Black-Eyed Pea Soup with Sweet Potatoes and Mustard Greens

Black-eyed peas offer the delicious earthiness of green peas but with a savory touch. If you don't like mustard greens or if you want to change up this recipe, you can use any fresh or frozen dark leafy greens you'd like. Julienned kale or collard greens are excellent choices and are equally rich in antioxidants.

Serves 10

- 1 tablespoon olive oil
- 1 medium yellow onion, peeled and chopped
- 2 medium stalks celery, chopped
- 1 large carrot, peeled and chopped
- 2 teaspoons salt
- 1 teaspoon dried thyme
- 2 teaspoons dried oregano
- 1 teaspoon ground cumin
- 1 dried chipotle chili, halved
- 2 bay leaves
- 1 pound dried black-eyed peas, washed and picked through for undesirables
- 2 quarts vegetable stock
- 1 large sweet potato, peeled and diced into 1" cubes
- 1 (10-ounce) package frozen mustard greens, chopped
- 1 (22-ounce) can diced tomatoes, drained
- ¼ teaspoon chopped fresh cilantro

1. In a large, heavy-bottomed Dutch oven, heat oil 1 minute over medium heat. Add onion, celery, carrot, and salt; cook 5 minutes until onions are translucent. Add thyme, oregano, cumin, chipotle chili, and bay leaves; cook additional 2 minutes.
2. Add black-eyed peas and vegetable stock. Bring to a boil over high heat, then simmer on low heat 2 hours, until beans are very tender.
3. Add sweet potato and cook 20 minutes. Stir in chopped mustard greens and tomatoes. Cook additional 10 minutes until potatoes and greens are tender. Adjust consistency with additional vegetable stock. The soup should have lots of broth.
4. Remove bay leaves. Serve garnished with chopped cilantro.

PER SERVING

Calories: 107 | Fat: 2.4g | Protein: 4.8g | Sodium: 1,283mg | Fiber: 5.2g | Carbohydrates: 18.6g | Net Carbohydrates: 13.4g | Sugar: 5.2g

Tuscan White Bean Soup

Beans are full of fiber, which not only keeps you regular but also keeps you full longer. This delicious Tuscan White Bean Soup will keep your hunger at bay.

Serves 8

2 tablespoons olive oil, divided

1 medium yellow onion, peeled and chopped

1 large leek, white part only, finely chopped

3 cloves garlic, peeled and finely chopped

3 teaspoons fresh chopped rosemary

1 bay leaf

3 quarts vegetable stock

2 cups large white beans soaked overnight

¼ teaspoon salt

¼ teaspoon ground white pepper

1. In a large soup pot over medium heat, heat 1 tablespoon olive oil 1 minute. Add onion, leek, and garlic; cook 10 minutes until onions are translucent, stirring frequently. Add rosemary and bay leaf; cook an additional 5 minutes.
2. Add stock and beans to pot. Bring to a full boil over high heat. Reduce heat to low, and cook 60 minutes until beans are very tender and starting to fall apart.
3. Remove bay leaf. Purée ⅔ of soup in a blender; add back to rest of soup. Season with salt and pepper.
4. Serve each bowl with equal amounts of the remaining 1 tablespoon of olive oil sprinkled on top.

PER SERVING

Calories: 237 | Fat: 5.1g | Protein: 15.4g | Sodium: 1,379mg | Fiber: 8.2g | Carbohydrates: 36.3g | Net Carbohydrates: 28.1g | Sugar: 3.2g

Vegan Chili

If you prefer a meaty chili, you can add some ground beef or ground turkey to this recipe by cooking the beef with the onions. With or without the meat, this hearty chili will keep you full (and satisfied!) for hours.

Serves 8

¼ cup olive oil

2 cups chopped peeled yellow onion

1 cup chopped peeled carrots

2 cups chopped seeded assorted bell peppers

2 teaspoons salt

4 teaspoons ground cumin

1 tablespoon chopped peeled garlic

2 medium jalapeños, stemmed, seeded, and chopped

1 tablespoon ground ancho chili pepper

1 chipotle in adobo, chopped

1 (28-ounce) can plum tomatoes, roughly chopped, juice included

3 (15.5-ounce) cans beans, drained and rinsed: 1 red kidney, 1 cannellini, and 1 black

1 cup tomato juice

2 tablespoons finely chopped peeled red onions

2 tablespoons chopped fresh cilantro

1. Heat oil in a large, heavy-bottomed Dutch oven or soup pot over medium heat 1 minute. Add onions, carrots, bell peppers, and salt; cook 15 minutes over medium heat until onions are soft.
2. In a small dry skillet over medium heat, toast cumin 1 minute. Add cumin to pot after toasted.
3. Add garlic, jalapeños, ancho, and chipotle to vegetable mixture; cook an additional 5 minutes.
4. Stir in tomatoes, beans, and tomato juice. Simmer covered 45 minutes over low heat.
5. Serve garnished with red onions and cilantro.

PER SERVING

Calories: 263 | Fat: 7.5g | Protein: 10.7g | Sodium: 1,188mg | Fiber: 12.6g | Carbohydrates: 41.0g | Net Carbohydrates: 28.4g | Sugar: 11.4g

Lamb Patties

The lamb can be served rare to medium-rare, but the egg should be thoroughly cooked. Fruit chutneys or chia seed jams are perfect complements to Lamb Patties.

Serves 2

1 medium shallot, peeled and minced
2 cloves garlic, peeled and minced
½ pound ground lamb
1 large egg white
¼ cup dried currants

¼ cup whole pistachio nuts
½ teaspoon ground cinnamon
¼ teaspoon freshly cracked black peppercorns
⅛ teaspoon salt

1. Preheat oven to 350°F.
2. In a medium bowl, mix all ingredients.
3. Form mixture into 6 small ovals. Place in an 8" × 8" baking dish and bake 15 minutes. Serve warm.

PER SERVING

Calories: 399 | Fat: 21.8g | Protein: 27.3g | Sodium: 243mg | Fiber: 3.6g | Carbohydrates: 21.4g | Net Carbohydrates: 17.8g | Sugar: 14.3g

Pork and Fennel Meatballs

These meatballs can be described as earthy and definitely tasty. Serve either as appetizers or as a full meal with pasta and marinara sauce with a sprinkle of chopped fresh parsley.

Makes 24 meatballs

1 pound 84 percent lean ground pork

2 tablespoons roughly chopped fresh flat-leaf parsley

3 tablespoons almond meal

1 large egg

¼ teaspoon salt

½ teaspoon freshly ground black pepper

1½ tablespoons olive oil

2 teaspoons fennel seeds

1. In a large mixing bowl, combine pork, parsley, almond meal, egg, salt, and pepper. Shape mixture into 24 (1") meatballs.
2. In a medium skillet, heat oil over medium heat 1 minute and sauté fennel seeds until fragrant, about 4 minutes.
3. Add meatballs to pan. Brown meatballs on all sides, about 20 minutes total. Meatballs are cooked through when no longer pink inside. Serve hot.

PER 1 MEATBALL

Calories: 54 | Fat: 4.1g | Protein: 3.9g | Sodium: 38mg | Fiber: 0.2g | Carbohydrates: 0.3g | Net Carbohydrates: 0.1g | Sugar: 0.0g

Mushroom Pork Medallions

These Mushroom Pork Medallions are gluten-free, Paleo-approved, and extremely delicious. The flax meal adds a rich, nutty flavor, as well as omega-3 fatty acids and antioxidants.

Serves 2

1 tablespoon olive oil

1 pound pork tenderloin, sliced into ½"-thick medallions

1 small yellow onion, peeled and sliced

¼ cup sliced white mushrooms

1 clove garlic, peeled and minced

2 teaspoons flax meal

½ cup no-salt-added beef broth

¼ teaspoon dried rosemary, crushed

⅛ teaspoon freshly ground black pepper

1. In a large skillet, heat olive oil over medium-high heat 30 seconds. Add pork and brown 2 minutes on each side. Remove pork from skillet and set aside.
2. In same skillet, add onions, mushrooms, and garlic and sauté 1 minute. Stir in flax meal until blended.
3. Gradually stir in broth, then add rosemary and pepper. Bring to a boil over high heat. Cook and stir 1 minute until thickened.
4. Lay pork medallions over mixture in skillet. Reduce heat to low; cover and simmer 15 minutes until meat juices run clear. Serve hot.

PER SERVING

Calories: 311 | Fat: 13.2g | Protein: 40.7g | Sodium: 433mg | Fiber: 1.3g | Carbohydrates: 5.8g | Net Carbohydrates: 4.5g | Sugar: 2.1g

Citrus Flank Steak

This citrusy steak pairs perfectly with a garden salad garnished with strawberries or blueberries.

Serves 6

¼ cup toasted sesame oil

1 tablespoon freshly squeezed lime juice

1 tablespoon pineapple juice

1 tablespoon pure maple syrup

1 (5") knob ginger, peeled and thinly sliced

¼ teaspoon salt

¼ teaspoon freshly ground black pepper

1 (1½-pound) flank steak

2 teaspoons olive oil

1. In a food processor, mix sesame oil, lime juice, pineapple juice, maple syrup, ginger, salt, and pepper until smooth, about 30 seconds; pour into a large bowl.
2. Add steak to bowl and cover with marinade. Refrigerate covered 4 hours.
3. Heat olive oil in a large cast-iron skillet over medium heat 1 minute, or heat grill to medium-high.
4. Cook steak in skillet or grill steak 8 minutes on each side. Transfer steak to a cutting board; cover loosely with foil and let rest 10 minutes.
5. Slice steak against the grain and serve.

PER SERVING

Calories: 333 | Fat: 27.5g | Protein: 16.3g | Sodium: 52mg | Fiber: 0.0g | Carbohydrates: 0.3g | Net Carbohydrates: 0.3g | Sugar: 0.2g

Filet Mignon Salad

Filet mignon, the most tender and popular cut of beef, is dressed to the nines in greens, tomatoes, and goat cheese in this filling salad.

Serves 2

¼ large head romaine lettuce (ribs removed), chopped

½ large head Belgian endive (about 1½ cups), trimmed and thinly sliced crosswise

¼ cup chopped fresh basil

1½ cups baby arugula

2 teaspoons pure maple syrup

½ cup rice wine vinegar

1½ tablespoons freshly squeezed lemon juice

½ teaspoon sea salt

½ teaspoon freshly ground black pepper

½ cup plus 1½ teaspoons olive oil, divided

1 tablespoon unsalted grass-fed butter

½ pound filet mignon

2 ounces crumbled goat cheese

8 cherry tomatoes, halved

1. In a large salad bowl combine romaine, endive, basil, and arugula.
2. In a food processor or blender, add maple syrup, vinegar, lemon juice, salt, and pepper. With machine running on low speed, slowly blend in ½ cup oil. Set aside.
3. Melt butter with remaining olive oil in a medium cast-iron skillet or stainless-steel skillet over medium heat 1 minute. Add filet mignon and cook 7 minutes on each side for medium-rare (or longer, depending on desired degree of doneness). Remove from heat and allow to stand 5 minutes. Slice into strips of medium thickness.
4. Add filet mignon, goat cheese, and cherry tomatoes to salad bowl. Pour in dressing. Toss well to coat, then serve.

PER SERVING

Calories: 910 | Fat: 77.1g | Protein: 36.6g | Sodium: 602mg | Fiber: 4.1g | Carbohydrates: 12.7g | Net Carbohydrates: 8.6g | Sugar: 7.5g

Beef with Spinach and Sweet Potatoes

This Beef with Spinach and Sweet Potatoes is a perfectly complete meal all in one. You'll enjoy a great balance of high-quality protein, vegetables, and carbohydrates. If potatoes start to stick while cooking, add more vinegar.

Serves 4

1 pound organic or grass-fed beef tenderloin, cut into 4 medallions
¼ teaspoon salt
¼ teaspoon freshly ground black pepper
3 teaspoons olive oil, divided
½ pound sweet potatoes, peeled and cut into ½" cubes
½ teaspoon ground turmeric
¼ teaspoon chili powder
2 tablespoons rice wine vinegar
3 tablespoons pure maple syrup
1½ cups fresh baby spinach
⅓ cup toasted pumpkin seeds

1. Season beef with salt and pepper. Heat 2 teaspoons oil in a 9" cast-iron skillet over medium-high heat 1 minute. Add beef to skillet and cook 3 minutes on each side for medium-rare. Transfer to plate and cover with foil.
2. Add remaining oil to skillet along with sweet potatoes. Cook over medium-high heat until browned, about 15 minutes. Stir in turmeric and chili powder and cook an additional 1 minute.
3. Add vinegar and maple syrup to skillet. Add spinach, ½ cup at a time, and cook 2 minutes, stirring.
4. Transfer spinach and sweet potatoes to plates and top with beef, followed by equal amounts of pumpkin seeds on each.

PER SERVING

Calories: 779 | Fat: 49.4g | Protein: 43.6g | Sodium: 487mg | Fiber: 5.7g | Carbohydrates: 31.0g | Net Carbohydrates: 25.3g | Sugar: 6.7g

Stuffed Peppers with Ground Turkey

These stuffed peppers store very well, so you can make them in advance. This recipe is also a basic template, so feel free to add any extra vegetables that you have on hand.

Serves 3

1 tablespoon olive oil
1 pound ground turkey
1 tablespoon garlic-infused oil, divided
2 medium Roma tomatoes, chopped
2 tablespoons pine nuts
1 cup cooked brown rice
1½ teaspoons chili powder
½ teaspoon ground cumin

1 teaspoon smoked paprika
3 tablespoons chopped fresh cilantro
3 large bell peppers (1 orange, 1 yellow, 1 green), stemmed, halved, and seeded
2 tablespoons coconut oil, melted
6 (1-ounce) slices goat cheese
3 tablespoons no-sugar-added salsa

1. Preheat oven to 375°F.
2. Heat olive oil in a large skillet over medium-high heat 1 minute. Add turkey and cook until browned, about 7 minutes.
3. Add half of garlic oil to skillet along with tomatoes and pine nuts; stir and heat through, about 3 minutes.
4. Add brown rice and stir to combine. Stir in remaining half of garlic oil, chili powder, cumin, paprika, and cilantro. Remove from heat.
5. Stuff halved peppers with brown rice mixture and brush outside of peppers with coconut oil. Place peppers in a 9" × 13" shallow baking dish. Top each pepper with a slice of goat cheese. Loosely cover dish with foil.
6. Bake 40 minutes until peppers are tender. Garnish with salsa and serve.

PER SERVING
Calories: 779 | Fat: 49.4g | Protein: 43.6g | Sodium: 487mg | Fiber: 5.7g | Carbohydrates: 31.0g | Net Carbohydrates: 25.3g | Sugar: 6.7g

Chicken Burgers

This basic recipe will become a staple for your intermittent fasting regimen. Chicken Burgers are easy to whip up and they store well, so you can always have a quick meal on the go. You can also make them your own by substituting any type of meat and spices.

Serves 4

1 pound ground chicken
½ teaspoon salt
½ teaspoon ground white pepper

1 large egg, beaten
¼ cup grated Parmesan cheese
1 tablespoon olive oil

1. In a large bowl, mix all ingredients except oil together with your hands until well combined.
2. Shape mixture into 4 patties.
3. In a large skillet heat oil on medium-high 1 minute and add burgers. Brown on one side about 5 minutes, then flip and cook other side another 5 minutes until cooked through. Serve hot.

PER SERVING

Calories: 224 | Fat: 13.9g | Protein: 21.9g | Sodium: 480mg | Fiber: 0.9g | Carbohydrates: 1.2g | Net Carbohydrates: 0.3g | Sugar: 0.1g

Slow Cooker Chicken Tagine

Tagine is a stew that originated in Morocco and is also found in other areas of North Africa. It's also known as tavas *in Cypriot cuisine. Enjoy this easier version of a more traditional tagine recipe!*

Serves 4

1½ tablespoons sweet paprika
1 teaspoon ground cinnamon
1½ tablespoons ground coriander
1½ teaspoons ground turmeric
2 teaspoons ground cardamom
1½ teaspoons ground allspice
⅛ teaspoon wheat-free asafetida powder
¼ teaspoon sea salt
¼ teaspoon freshly ground black pepper
4 (5-ounce) skinless, boneless

chicken thighs, halved
1 tablespoon olive oil
1½ teaspoons ground ginger
1½ teaspoons saffron
1 (14-ounce) can whole tomatoes, drained
⅓ cup canned chickpeas, thoroughly drained and rinsed
1 quart chicken stock
1 lemon, chopped into wedges
1 tablespoon chopped fresh flat-leaf parsley

1. In a small skillet over medium heat, toast paprika, cinnamon, coriander, turmeric, cardamom, and allspice until fragrant, about 2 minutes. Set aside and allow to cool 3 minutes.
2. Once cooled, sprinkle spice mixture, asafetida, salt, and pepper on both sides of each halved chicken thigh.
3. In a large skillet, heat oil over medium heat 1 minute. Add chicken thighs and sear until browned, about 2 minutes on each side. Remove from heat and place chicken in a 4- to 6-quart slow cooker.
4. Add ginger to small skillet. Cook over medium heat and stir 2 minutes, then add to slow cooker.
5. Add saffron, tomatoes, chickpeas, and chicken stock to slow cooker. Cook on high 4 hours. Once done, remove to serving dish and garnish with lemon and parsley.

PER SERVING

Calories: 381 | Fat: 15.8g | Protein: 34.2g | Sodium: 810mg | Fiber: 3.8g | Carbohydrates: 21.5g | Net Carbohydrates: 17.7g | Sugar: 9.4g

Lemon Thyme Chicken

Lemon and thyme pair together to make this delicious citrus chicken—but it's not just flavor that thyme offers. This herb has also been shown to help lower blood pressure and cholesterol levels and may even improve your mood.

Serves 4

4 skin-on chicken thighs and 4 skin-on chicken drumsticks (approximately ½ pound of each)

3 medium lemons, halved

Zest of 1 medium lemon

1 tablespoon unsalted grass-fed butter, melted

¼ teaspoon sea salt

½ teaspoon freshly ground black pepper

2 tablespoons fresh thyme leaves

6 fresh basil leaves, torn

1. Preheat oven to 375°F.
2. In a large bowl, add chicken. Squeeze juice from lemons into bowl.
3. Add lemon zest, butter, salt, pepper, and thyme; toss well with your hands. Place chicken in a 9" × 13" baking dish.
4. Bake chicken 40 minutes, basting every 10 minutes. Skin should get crispy and meat should be cooked through.
5. Garnish with basil leaves and serve.

PER SERVING

Calories: 480 | Fat: 22.5g | Protein: 58.6g | Sodium: 380mg | Fiber: 0.5g | Carbohydrates: 2.3g | Net Carbohydrates: 1.8g | Sugar: 0.6g

Spinach and Feta–Stuffed Chicken Breasts

This recipe is easy to make and requires only a few ingredients. You'll be just 30 minutes away from a delicious meal when it's time to break your fast.

Serves 2

1 tablespoon garlic-infused olive oil
1 cup fresh spinach leaves
½ cup crumbled feta cheese
2 (4-ounce) boneless, skinless
chicken breasts, pounded to ¼"
thickness

1 large egg, lightly beaten
1 cup almond meal

1. Preheat oven to 350°F.
2. Heat oil in a medium skillet over low heat 1 minute. Cook spinach until soft, about 3 minutes. Add feta, stir a few times, and remove from heat.
3. Place half of spinach mixture on each chicken breast. Wrap chicken around mixture and secure with toothpicks.
4. In a shallow bowl, add egg. In a separate shallow bowl, add almond meal. Roll each breast in egg, tap off any excess, then roll in almond meal until well coated.
5. Place chicken in an 8" × 8" casserole dish. Bake 30 minutes and serve.

PER SERVING

Calories: 395 | Fat: 24.1g | Protein: 35.8g | Sodium: 423mg | Fiber: 1.8g | Carbohydrates: 5.2g | Net Carbohydrates: 3.4g | Sugar: 2.1g

Salmon with Herbs

Salmon is one of the best fatty fish to consume because it's rich in omega-3 fatty acids and doesn't contain a lot of mercury like bigger fish do. However, you can tweak this recipe and use any fish that you like.

Serves 4

1 (1-pound) salmon fillet
¼ teaspoon salt
½ teaspoon freshly ground black
  pepper
¼ cup plus 2 tablespoons olive oil
¼ cup chopped fresh dill

2 tablespoons roughly chopped
  fresh rosemary
¼ cup fresh flat-leaf parsley
2 tablespoons fresh thyme leaves
2 tablespoons freshly squeezed
  lemon juice

1. Preheat oven to 250°F.
2. Coat a 9" × 13" baking dish with cooking spray. Lay salmon skin side down and sprinkle with salt and pepper.
3. Blend olive oil with dill, rosemary, parsley, thyme, and lemon juice in a small food processor, about 15 seconds. Use a spatula or your hands to pat herb paste over salmon.
4. Bake salmon 22–28 minutes depending on thickness. Insert tines of a fork into thickest part of fillet and gently pull. If fish flakes easily, it is done.
5. Slide a spatula under fish and set on a cutting board. Cut into equal pieces and serve.

PER SERVING

Calories: 342 | Fat: 26.2g | Protein: 22.8g | Sodium: 197mg | Fiber: 0.5g | Carbohydrates: 1.5g | Net Carbohydrates: 1.0g | Sugar: 0.2g

Mediterranean Flaky Fish with Vegetables

The lovely flavors of the Mediterranean are paired with flaky fish in this recipe, creating a healthy and tasty dinner. Serve with a salad and potatoes.

Serves 4

4 (3.5-ounce) skinless Atlantic cod fillets
1 cup grated zucchini
¼ cup thinly sliced fresh basil, plus 4 whole basil leaves, divided
20 cherry tomatoes, halved
10 black olives, sliced
¼ teaspoon salt
½ teaspoon freshly ground black pepper
4 tablespoons dry white wine
4 tablespoons olive oil

1. Preheat oven to 400°F.
2. To make parchment pockets: Cut a 17" × 11" piece of parchment paper. With one longer edge closest to you, fold in half from left to right. Using scissors, cut out a large heart shape, using the fold as the center of the heart and cutting half of a heart shape. Repeat to cut four hearts in all. On a large cutting board, lay down one parchment heart and place fish on half of heart, leaving at least a 1½" border around fillet. Repeat with remaining fish fillets. Lay parchment hearts in a 9" × 13" baking dish.
3. In a medium bowl, combine zucchini, sliced basil, tomatoes, olives, salt, and pepper. Stir to combine.
4. Evenly distribute vegetable mixture over each fish fillet on parchment hearts.
5. Take free side of each parchment heart and fold over fish, making both edges of the heart line up. Starting at rounded end, crimp and fold edges together tightly. Leave a few inches at pointed end unfolded. Grab pointed edge and tilt heart to pour in 1 tablespoon each of wine and oil. Repeat for each heart. Finish by crimping edges and twisting pointed ends around and under pockets.
6. Bake fish until just cooked through, about 12 minutes. Poke a tooth pick through parchment paper. Fish should be done if toothpick easily slides through fish. Carefully cut open packets (steam will escape). Garnish with whole basil leaves and serve.

PER SERVING
Calories: 230 | Fat: 14.8g | Protein: 16.5g | Sodium: 533mg | Fiber: 1.8g | Carbohydrates: 5.5g | Net Carbohydrates: 3.7g | Sugar: 3.1g

Basic Baked Scallops

This yummy seafood recipe takes less than 30 minutes to make and pairs well with green beans or a side salad.

Serves 2

¾ pound sea scallops

2 tablespoons freshly squeezed lemon juice

2½ tablespoons unsalted grass-fed butter, melted

¼ teaspoon sea salt

½ teaspoon freshly ground black pepper

2 tablespoons chopped fresh flat-leaf parsley

½ cup almond meal

½ teaspoon smoked paprika

2 tablespoons olive oil

1. Preheat oven to 425°F.
2. Toss together scallops, lemon juice, butter, salt, and pepper in a 2-quart baking dish.
3. In a medium bowl, combine parsley, almond meal, paprika, and olive oil. Sprinkle mixture on top of scallops.
4. Bake scallops 14 minutes until they are heated through and almond meal is golden. Serve immediately.

PER SERVING

Calories: 540 | Fat: 42.7g | Protein: 26.8g | Sodium: 907mg | Fiber: 3.5g | Carbohydrates: 13.4g | Net Carbohydrates: 9.9g | Sugar: 1.5g

Fish Curry

The salmon in this Fish Curry provides a healthy dose of omega-3 fatty acids that can help you fight inflammation and keep your brain healthy.

Serves 2

1 medium carrot, peeled and chopped

2 cups chicken broth

¼ teaspoon gluten-free fish sauce

1 (13.5-ounce) can unsweetened full-fat coconut milk, refrigerated overnight, cream only

1 medium Roma tomato, diced

½ small stalk celery, diced

1 tablespoon curry powder

¼ teaspoon ground cumin

¼ teaspoon ground coriander

½ teaspoon ground turmeric

¼ teaspoon freshly grated ginger

2 tablespoons roughly chopped fresh cilantro

½ pound wild-caught salmon, skin removed

1. Boil carrots in a medium saucepan over high heat until softened just slightly, about 3 minutes. Drain, discarding water, and add chicken broth and fish sauce to pan.
2. Add coconut cream, tomato, celery, curry powder, cumin, coriander, and turmeric to pan.
3. Bring to a boil over high heat; cover, reduce heat to low, and simmer 20 minutes, stirring every 5 minutes.
4. Stir in ginger and cilantro. Add fish and stir to cover with liquid.
5. Cook 5 minutes over medium heat to achieve flaky fish, then serve.

PER SERVING

Calories: 592 | Fat: 45.5g | Protein: 29.7g | Sodium: 1,086mg | Fiber: 3.8g | Carbohydrates: 15.2g | Net Carbohydrates: 11.4g | Sugar: 5.1g

Lentil-Stuffed Peppers

These Lentil-Stuffed Peppers are even better as leftovers. Make them in advance and store them in your refrigerator for a quick meal that's ready to eat when you're ready to break your fast.

Serves 6

1 tablespoon olive oil
2 medium yellow onions, peeled and finely diced
2 medium stalks celery, finely diced
2 large carrots, peeled and finely diced
4 cups vegetable stock, divided
3 cups dried red lentils

6 medium red bell peppers, tops cut off and set aside, seeds and ribs removed
6 sprigs fresh oregano, tops reserved and remaining leaves chopped
3 ounces feta cheese
¼ teaspoon freshly cracked black peppercorns

1. Heat oil in a large saucepot over medium heat 1 minute. Add onions, celery, and carrots; sauté 5 minutes, then add 1 cup vegetable stock and lentils. Simmer 20 minutes until lentils are fully cooked.
2. Place bell peppers in a large, shallow pot with remaining 3 cups vegetable stock. Cover and simmer over medium heat 10 minutes, then remove from heat.
3. In a large bowl, mix together lentil mixture, chopped oregano, feta, and black peppercorns; spoon mixture into bell peppers.
4. Serve peppers with stem tops ajar. Garnish with reserved oregano tops.

PER SERVING

Calories: 473 | Fat: 7.8g | Protein: 28.3g | Sodium: 745mg | Fiber: 14.3g | Carbohydrates: 75.3g | Net Carbohydrates: 61.0g | Sugar: 8.7g

Marinated London Broil

Cinnamon and cloves may not be your first thought when it comes to steak rubs, but these spices bring out mouthwatering flavors. After cooking, cut the London broil against the grain.

Serves 6

1 cup dry red wine
1 tablespoon olive oil
1 teaspoon ground cinnamon
½ teaspoon ground cloves
1 teaspoon ground cumin

¼ teaspoon freshly cracked black peppercorns
¼ teaspoon salt
1½ pounds London broil

1. Preheat grill to medium heat.
2. In a small bowl, mix together wine, oil, and seasonings. Coat meat in mixture, then grill to desired doneness. Slice and serve.

PER SERVING
Calories: 170 | Fat: 5.7g | Protein: 24.6g | Sodium: 159mg | Fiber: 0.4g | Carbohydrates: 1.0g | Net Carbohydrates: 0.6g | Sugar: 0.1g

Not Your Grandmother's Eggplant Parmigiana

This eggplant parmigiana has all the flavor of your grandmother's recipe but with a healthier twist. The coconut flour and almond meal give the eggplant a nice breading while making this recipe gluten-free.

Serves 4

3 large eggs, beaten
½ cup water
1 cup coconut flour
3 cups almond meal
1 medium eggplant (about 1 pound), thinly sliced
¼ cup olive oil, divided

1 (24-ounce) jar no-sugar-added tomato sauce
1 pound shredded part-skim mozzarella cheese
1 teaspoon chopped fresh flat-leaf parsley

1. In a medium shallow bowl, mix eggs with water. In a second medium shallow bowl, add flour. In a third medium shallow bowl, add almond meal.
2. Dip both sides of one eggplant slice in flour and shake off excess, then dip both sides of slice in egg mixture and shake off excess, and then dip both sides of slice in almond meal and shake off excess. Set aside. Repeat process with remaining eggplant slices.
3. Preheat oven to 350°F.
4. Heat 2 tablespoons oil in a heavy medium skillet over medium heat 1 minute.
5. Fry slices in hot skillet over medium-high heat until golden (about 3 minutes per slice, 1½ minutes per side), adding remaining oil as needed. Drain fried eggplant on a rack or paper towels.
6. Line eggplant slices in a 9" × 13" baking dish. Top each slice with 1 tablespoon tomato sauce and 1 small mound shredded cheese. Bake until cheese is melted, browning, and bubbly, about 15 minutes.
7. Serve garnished with chopped parsley, with remaining tomato sauce on the side.

PER SERVING

Calories: 680 | Fat: 41.9g | Protein: 42.5g | Sodium: 1,672mg | Fiber: 16.3g | Carbohydrates: 34.7g | Net Carbohydrates: 18.4g | Sugar: 14.1g

Artichoke Dip

This Artichoke Dip is a lighter version of the original but with all the same delicious flavor. You can serve it alongside your favorite vegetables or gluten-free crackers.

Serves 8

2 (14-ounce) cans quartered artichoke hearts, drained, rinsed, and chopped

1 medium red bell pepper, stemmed, seeded, and finely chopped

1 medium green bell pepper, stemmed, seeded, and finely chopped

3 cloves garlic, peeled and minced

2 cups homemade mayonnaise

¼ teaspoon ground white pepper

1 pound grated Parmesan cheese, divided

1. Preheat oven to 325°F.
2. In a large bowl, mix all ingredients except ¼ pound Parmesan cheese. Spread mixture in a 9" × 9" baking dish and sprinkle remaining Parmesan on top.
3. Bake 45 minutes until golden brown. Serve hot.

PER SERVING

Calories: 643 | Fat: 53.9g | Protein: 17.8g | Sodium: 1,616mg | Fiber: 2.1g | Carbohydrates: 14.0g | Net Carbohydrates: 11.9g | Sugar: 12.3g

Curry Dip

The jalapeños in this dip give it a little bit of a kick, but if you prefer it less spicy, you can omit them or use finely diced green peppers in their place.

Makes 2½ cups

1 teaspoon olive oil
½ cup finely chopped peeled yellow onion
½ medium jalapeño, stemmed, seeded, and finely chopped (about 1 teaspoon)
2 teaspoons finely chopped seeded red bell pepper
1 teaspoon curry powder
1 teaspoon ground cumin
½ teaspoon ground coriander
½ teaspoon ground turmeric
⅛ teaspoon cayenne pepper
¼ teaspoon salt
1 tablespoon soft raisins
1 tablespoon water
1½ cups mayonnaise
1 tablespoon chopped fresh cilantro
⅛ teaspoon freshly squeezed lemon juice

1. Heat oil 30 seconds in a small skillet over medium heat. Add onion, jalapeño, and red bell pepper; cook 5 minutes, stirring occasionally until onions are translucent. Add curry powder, cumin, coriander, turmeric, cayenne pepper, and salt. Cook an additional minute until spices are very fragrant. Add raisins and water.
2. Transfer mixture to a food processor. Chop on high speed 30 seconds. Scrape down sides of bowl with a rubber spatula. Add mayonnaise and cilantro; process an additional 30 seconds until smooth and even. Add lemon juice and serve.

PER ½ CUP

Calories: 174 | Fat: 17.2g | Protein: 0.7g | Sodium: 257mg | Fiber: 0.8g | Carbohydrates: 4.2g | Net Carbohydrates: 3.4g | Sugar: 2.2g

What Is Curry Powder?

What we know as curry powder is actually a blend of spices, invented by the British to resemble one of the famous masalas (spice blends) of India. Most authentic Indian recipes call not for curry powder but a combination of spices (a masala) specifically designed for that dish.

Roasted Beets

Roasting brings natural juices to the surface of these magenta roots and caramelizes them into a sweet, intensely flavored crust. Snacking on beets can curb sugar cravings, so you're less likely to indulge in unhealthy foods during your feeding window.

Serves 8

2 pounds (about 8 large) beets, cut into 1" wedges

1 tablespoon olive oil

¼ teaspoon ground cinnamon

¼ teaspoon salt

¼ teaspoon chopped fresh flat-leaf parsley

1. Preheat oven to 350°F.
2. In a large bowl, toss beets with olive oil, cinnamon, and salt. Spread into a single layer on a nonstick baking sheet.
3. Roast on middle rack of oven until beets are tender, about 1 hour, turning once after 30 minutes. Serve hot, sprinkled with chopped parsley.

PER SERVING

Calories: 52 | Fat: 1.7g | Protein: 1.4g | Sodium: 139mg | Fiber: 2.5g | Carbohydrates: 8.3g | Net Carbohydrates: 5.8g | Sugar: 5.8g

Mushroom-Stuffed Tomatoes

Use any kind of ripe tomatoes you prefer for this dish. Late in the season, Roma tomatoes are usually the best choice since they keep a long time even when ripe. If using a processor to chop the mushrooms, "pulse" them in small batches, stopping before they clump.

Serves 6

4 medium shallots, peeled and finely chopped
2 tablespoons olive oil, divided
1 pound white mushrooms, finely chopped
1¼ teaspoons salt, divided
¼ cup white wine
¼ cup finely chopped fresh flat-leaf parsley
¼ teaspoon freshly ground black pepper
6 large ripe Roma tomatoes, halved crosswise, rounded ends trimmed flat
3 tablespoons almond meal

1. Preheat oven to 350°F.
2. Sauté shallots with 1 tablespoon olive oil 1 minute in a large skillet over medium heat. Add mushrooms and 1 teaspoon salt and raise heat to high. Cook, stirring occasionally, about 5 minutes, until mushrooms have given up their water and most water has evaporated.
3. Add white wine to skillet and cook an additional 5 minutes until wine has mostly evaporated. Stir in parsley, remove from heat, and season with pepper.
4. Scoop innards from tomatoes and season tomato cups with remaining salt. Fill each tomato with mushroom filling so that it mounds slightly, topping each mound with a sprinkle of almond meal.
5. Place stuffed tomatoes in a 9" × 13" baking dish and drizzle with remaining olive oil. Bake 25 minutes until soft. Serve hot.

PER SERVING
Calories: 106 | Fat: 6.4g | Protein: 4.2g | Sodium: 495mg | Fiber: 2.7g | Carbohydrates: 9.3g | Net Carbohydrates: 6.6g | Sugar: 5.1g

Onion Jam

The concentrated sweetness and naturally complex flavor of this caramelized onion spread come from slow cooking, which breaks down the cell walls of the onions, releasing 100 percent of their flavor. Serve it with gluten-free crackers.

Serves 8

2 tablespoons olive oil

2 sprigs fresh thyme, stems removed

8 large white onions, peeled, halved, and sliced thinly across the grain

½ teaspoon salt

1. Heat oil in a large heavy-bottomed Dutch oven over medium heat 1 minute until oil shimmers but does not smoke. Add thyme and sliced onions. Sprinkle with salt.
2. Reduce heat to low; cook slowly, stirring gently with a wooden spoon. As onions begin to caramelize (turn brown), use the wooden spoon to scrape dried-on juices from the bottom of the pot; stir regularly to incorporate as much of these browned juices as possible. Cook this way until onions are dark brown and mostly disintegrated into a thick spread, about 40 minutes total.
3. Remove from heat and cool to room temperature, or serve warm.

PER SERVING

Calories: 89 | Fat: 3.4g | Protein: 1.7g | Sodium: 151mg | Fiber: 2.6g | Carbohydrates: 14.0g | Net Carbohydrates: 11.4g | Sugar: 6.4g

Stuffed Eggs

These Stuffed Eggs are a variation on deviled eggs and make a great first course or garnish for a main-course salad. Their tops are attractively browned under the broiler.

Serves 8

8 large hard-boiled eggs, peeled and halved lengthwise
¼ cup Dijon mustard
3 tablespoons unsweetened full-fat coconut milk
2 tablespoons finely chopped shallots

1 tablespoon rice wine vinegar
1 tablespoon chopped fresh chives
1 tablespoon chopped fresh tarragon
¼ teaspoon salt
¼ teaspoon ground white pepper
¼ cup unsalted grass-fed butter

1. Turn on oven broiler to low.
2. Remove egg yolks from whites and combine yolks with mustard, milk, shallots, vinegar, chives, and tarragon in a medium bowl. Season with salt and pepper. Transfer mixture to a piping bag and pipe into egg whites (you can also use a spoon).
3. Place filled eggs in a 9" × 13" baking dish. Dot tops with butter and broil until tops are lightly browned, about 5 minutes. Serve warm.

PER SERVING

Calories: 161 | Fat: 12.3g | Protein: 7.1g | Sodium: 340mg | Fiber: 0.1g | Carbohydrates: 1.9g | Net Carbohydrates: 1.8g | Sugar: 0.8g

Cranberry Almond Granola

This Cranberry Almond Granola makes a delicious snack all on its own, but you can make it a meal by throwing it on top of some coconut-milk yogurt or pouring coconut or almond milk on top and garnishing with sliced banana.

Makes 2½ cups

1 tablespoon whole walnuts
1 tablespoon flaxseeds
1 cup gluten-free rolled oats
1 tablespoon slivered almonds
½ teaspoon ground cinnamon
3 tablespoons coconut oil, melted
3 tablespoons pure maple syrup

¼ teaspoon alcohol-free vanilla extract
¼ teaspoon alcohol-free almond extract
2 tablespoons no-sugar-added dried cranberries

1. Preheat oven to 350°F.
2. Using a food processor or blender, pulse walnuts until ground, about 5 seconds. Transfer walnuts to a large bowl. Next add flaxseeds to processor and pulse until finely ground, about 10 seconds. Transfer to large bowl with walnuts. Add oats, almonds, and cinnamon to bowl. Stir to combine.
3. In a small bowl, stir together oil, maple syrup, vanilla extract, and almond extract. Pour over oat mixture in large bowl and combine.
4. Spread granola on a rimmed, ungreased baking sheet and bake 15 minutes. Stir occasionally to ensure granola turns a light brown color.
5. Remove from oven and add cranberries, stirring to combine. Serve warm. Store in an airtight container in the refrigerator up to 3 weeks.

PER ¼ CUP
Calories: 105 | Fat: 5.8g | Protein: 1.9g | Sodium: 1mg | Fiber: 1.6g | Carbohydrates: 11.4g | Net Carbohydrates: 9.8g | Sugar: 4.0g

Mini Baked Eggplant Pizza Bites

These Mini Baked Eggplant Pizza Bites give you all the flavor of pizza with significantly more nutrients—and no gluten. They make a great grab-and-go snack or a mini meal all on their own.

Serves 4

2 medium eggplants, top and bottom ends cut off, cut into round slices, approximately ¼" thick
½ teaspoon salt
2 large eggs, beaten

¾ cup almond meal
2 tablespoons dried oregano
2 tablespoons olive oil
½ cup marinara sauce
¼ cup shredded mozzarella cheese

1. Preheat oven to 400°F.
2. Cut off sides of eggplant circles to make square shapes. Place slices in a colander and toss with salt. Let sit 10 minutes, then rinse with water.
3. In a small shallow bowl, add eggs. In a second small shallow bowl, add almond meal and oregano, stirring well to combine. Dredge eggplant squares in eggs, tap off any excess, and then dredge in almond meal. Place slices on one or two nonstick baking sheets.
4. Slowly drizzle olive oil to cover the top of each square. Bake 12 minutes.
5. Remove baking sheet from oven and spoon marinara sauce onto the center of each square, leaving edges of eggplant uncovered. Sprinkle mozzarella on top of squares. Bake an additional 3 minutes until cheese has melted. Serve hot.

PER SERVING

Calories: 247 | Fat: 16.5g | Protein: 9.0g | Sodium: 322mg | Fiber: 9.3g | Carbohydrates: 19.5g | Net Carbohydrates: 10.2g | Sugar: 11.2g

Quinoa Pizza Muffins

These Quinoa Pizza Muffins are a healthier, gluten-free twist on the classic fan favorite: English muffin pizzas. They'll satisfy your cravings for pizza with an added dose of nostalgia.

Makes 12 muffins

1 cup uncooked quinoa, rinsed
2 cups water
2 large eggs, beaten
1½ cups shredded mozzarella
  cheese
½ cup chopped fresh spinach
¼ cup chopped fresh basil

1 teaspoon dried oregano
½ teaspoon salt
½ teaspoon freshly ground black
  pepper
1½ cups no-sugar-added marinara
  sauce

1. In a medium saucepan, combine quinoa with water. Bring to a boil over high heat. Reduce heat to low, cover, and simmer until quinoa is tender, about 15 minutes.
2. Preheat oven to 350°F. Grease a 12-cup muffin tin with cooking spray.
3. In saucepan with quinoa, combine eggs, cheese, spinach, basil, oregano, salt, and pepper.
4. Add ¼ cup mixture to each muffin well. Press down gently on mixture with back of a spoon or with your fingers.
5. Bake 20 minutes. Allow to cool 5 minutes and serve topped with warmed marinara sauce.

PER 1 MUFFIN

Calories: 119 | Fat: 4.4g | Protein: 6.7g | Sodium: 278mg | Fiber: 1.6g | Carbohydrates: 12.1g | Net Carbohydrates: 10.5g | Sugar: 1.7g

Raspberry Lemon Chia Seed Jam

This jam is delicious on a warm scone, on gluten-free toast with butter, or mixed into a container of grass-fed or coconut-milk yogurt.

Makes 1 cup

½ pint (6 ounces) fresh raspberries
1 tablespoon freshly squeezed
  lemon juice
1 tablespoon lemon zest
2½ tablespoons pure maple syrup
1 tablespoon chia seeds

1. Add raspberries, lemon juice, lemon zest, and maple syrup to a small saucepan over medium-high heat. Cover. Stir occasionally until fruit begins to thicken, about 10 minutes.
2. Uncover and bring mixture to a boil over high heat (stirring often) until it reaches a sauce-like consistency, about 5 minutes.
3. Stir in chia seeds and cook, uncovered, an additional 2 minutes. Stir and remove from heat.
4. After jam has cooled, transfer to an airtight jar and refrigerate 3 hours before use. Jam will continue to thicken and can be refrigerated up to 2 weeks or frozen up to 2 months.

PER 2 TABLESPOONS
Calories: 34 | Fat: 0.5g | Protein: 0.5g | Sodium: 1mg | Fiber: 1.9g |
Carbohydrates: 7.5g | Net Carbohydrates: 5.6g | Sugar: 4.8g

Baked Apples

These Baked Apples satisfy a sweet craving without any added sweeteners. Leave the skin on the apples for extra fiber.

Serves 6

6 large Pink Lady apples, cores removed to ½" of bottom of apples

1 cup shredded unsweetened coconut

1 teaspoon ground cinnamon

1. Preheat oven to 350°F.
2. Place apples in a medium baking dish. Fill each apple center with coconut and sprinkle with cinnamon.
3. Bake 15 minutes. Apples are done when they are completely soft and brown on top. Serve hot.

PER SERVING

Calories: 203 | Fat: 8.0g | Protein: 1.4g | Sodium: 2mg | Fiber: 7.5g | Carbohydrates: 31.3g | Net Carbohydrates: 23.8g | Sugar: 21.6g

Cranberry Chutney

This Cranberry Chutney is a satisfying treat on its own, but it also makes a great topping for Chocolate Mug Cake (see recipe in this chapter).

Serves 2

2 cups fresh or frozen cranberries
¼ cup finely diced peeled red onion
1 cup coconut sugar

6 whole cloves
¼ cup water

Combine all ingredients in a small heavy-bottomed saucepot. Simmer on low heat 15 minutes until all cranberries are broken and have a saucy consistency. Remove from heat. Serve hot.

PER SERVING

Calories: 414 | Fat: 0.1g | Protein: 0.6g | Sodium: 2mg | Fiber: 4.9g | Carbohydrates: 110.1g | Net Carbohydrates: 105.2g | Sugar: 100.9g

Chocolate Mug Cake

You can make this Chocolate Mug Cake lower in carbohydrates by replacing the maple syrup with stevia or monk fruit.

Serves 1

¼ cup almond flour
1 tablespoon raw unsweetened cacao powder
1½ tablespoons maple syrup
1 teaspoon unsweetened full-fat coconut milk

1 teaspoon coconut oil
1 teaspoon vanilla extract
1 large egg

1. Combine all ingredients in a large mug and whisk with a fork to combine.
2. Microwave 90 seconds until a toothpick inserted in center comes out clean.
3. Serve immediately.

PER SERVING
Calories: 388 | Fat: 24.0g | Protein: 13.4g | Sodium: 74mg | Fiber: 4.0g | Carbohydrates: 30.0g | Net Carbohydrates: 26.0g | Sugar: 19.9g

Raspberry Lemon Oatmeal Bars

These Raspberry Lemon Oatmeal Bars are sweet enough to satisfy a dessert craving but also healthy enough to eat for breakfast. Double the recipe and store some in the freezer. You can thaw them out and have a quick breakfast ready to go when it's time to break your fast.

Serves 12

½ teaspoon coconut sugar

1¼ cups unsweetened almond milk

½ teaspoon alcohol-free vanilla extract

1 large egg

¼ cup pure maple syrup

3½ cups gluten-free quick-cooking oats

2 tablespoons freshly squeezed lemon juice

2 cups fresh raspberries

1. Preheat oven to 350°F.
2. In a large bowl, whisk together sugar, milk, vanilla, egg, and maple syrup. Add oats, lemon juice, and raspberries. Stir well to combine.
3. Pour mixture into a 9" × 13" baking dish greased with butter and bake 25 minutes.
4. Allow to cool 1 hour, then cut into 12 small rectangles. Refrigerate in an airtight container until ready to serve, up to 3 days. Serve warm.

PER SERVING

Calories: 143 | Fat: 2.5g | Protein: 5.0g | Sodium: 25mg | Fiber: 4.4g | Carbohydrates: 24.4g | Net Carbohydrates: 20.0g | Sugar: 5.8g

Peanut Butter Cookies

These cookies are very easy and quick to make and use minimal, natural ingredients. Make them in advance and store them for a quick dessert that you can eat before your feeding window ends.

Makes 18 cookies

1 cup all-natural no-sugar-added peanut butter

1 cup coconut sugar

1 teaspoon alcohol-free vanilla extract

1 tablespoon pure maple syrup

1 large egg

½ teaspoon sea salt

1. Preheat oven to 350°F.
2. In a medium bowl, mix together peanut butter, sugar, vanilla, maple syrup, and egg.
3. Spoon out 1 tablespoon dough for each cookie, form into a ball, and place about 1" apart on an ungreased baking sheet. Use prongs of a fork to gently press down and flatten cookies. Turn fork and press down again to make a crosshatch pattern. Lightly sprinkle salt on top of cookies.
4. Bake 5 minutes, then turn baking sheet 180 degrees and continue baking another 5 minutes. Cookies should be golden brown around the edges. Cool 10 minutes before serving.

PER 1 COOKIE

Calories: 136 | Fat: 7.8g | Protein: 3.9g | Sodium: 47mg | Fiber: 0.9g | Carbohydrates: 13.2g | Net Carbohydrates: 12.3g | Sugar: 11.8g

Peach Tart

When peaches are in season, this scrumptious dessert is a must-make item.

Serves 8

4 cups sliced peeled and cored
fresh peaches

¼ cup coconut sugar

1 tablespoon freshly squeezed
lemon juice

1 prepared piecrust

1. In a large mixing bowl, combine peaches, sugar, and lemon juice and toss to coat.
2. Pour peaches into prepared pie shell and refrigerate 5 hours or up to overnight before serving.

PER SERVING

Calories: 773 | Fat: 73.7g | Protein: 6.0g | Sodium: 2mg | Fiber: 6.8g | Carbohydrates: 25.7g | Net Carbohydrates: 18.9g | Sugar: 18.0g

Frozen: The Next Best Thing

If you're making a fruit recipe, you don't always have to wait until the fruit you crave is in season. Manufacturers have perfected the art of flash-freezing fruits at their peak to preserve the nutrients and vitamins.

Fruit Salad with Ginger and Lemon Juice

Traditional fruit salad is a few fruits and melons thrown together and served. This recipe includes a tasty dressing of freshly squeezed lemon juice and minced ginger for a heightened flavor experience that will make fruit salad mean something completely new.

Serves 2

1 medium grapefruit, peeled, seeded, and sectioned

1 cup pineapple chunks

1 cup green seedless grapes, sliced

1 medium Granny Smith apple, cored and chopped

1 cup cubed, peeled, and seeded cantaloupe

1 cup cubed, peeled, and seeded honeydew melon

3 tablespoons freshly squeezed lemon juice

2 tablespoons peeled and freshly grated ginger

½ cup shredded unsweetened coconut

¼ cup raw cacao nibs

1. In a large mixing bowl, combine fruit, lemon juice, ginger, coconut, and cacao nibs. Toss to coat.
2. Divide salad between two salad bowls and serve.

PER SERVING

Calories: 459 | Fat: 17.9g | Protein: 5.0g | Sodium: 46mg | Fiber: 14.3g | Carbohydrates: 74.1g | Net Carbohydrates: 59.8g | Sugar: 44.5g

Appendix: Best Food Choices

Getting to a healthier lifestyle means making good choices about the food you eat. Here is a list of the healthiest alternatives for each of the major food groups.

Meat, Poultry, and Eggs

Choose organic whenever possible:

- Bison
- Elk
- Grass-fed beef
- Grass-fed lamb
- Pasture-raised chicken
- Pasture-raised duck
- Pasture-raised eggs
- Pasture-raised pork
- Venison

Seafood

- Anchovies
- Clams
- Herring
- Mackerel
- Mussels
- Oysters
- Sardines
- Scallops
- Shrimp
- Wild-caught salmon

Grains and Legumes

- Adzuki beans
- Amaranth
- Black beans
- Black-eyed peas
- Brown rice
- Buckwheat
- Garbanzo beans (chickpeas)
- Lentils
- Millet
- Mung beans
- Peas
- Quinoa
- Sorghum
- Teff
- White beans
- Wild rice

Fruits and Vegetables

The following is the Environmental Working Group's Dirty Dozen list (in descending order), included to let you know to choose organic versions of these whenever possible:

- Strawberries
- Spinach
- Nectarines
- Apples
- Grapes
- Peaches

- Cherries
- Pears
- Tomatoes
- Celery
- Potatoes
- Sweet bell peppers

- Monk fruit
- Palm sugar
- Pure maple syrup
- Raw honey
- Stevia (sparingly)

The Environmental Working Group's Clean Fifteen list of conventional produce (beginning with the cleanest):

- Avocados
- Sweet corn
- Pineapples
- Cabbages
- Onions
- Frozen sweet peas
- Papayas
- Asparagus
- Mangoes
- Eggplants
- Honeydew melons
- Kiwis
- Cantaloupes
- Cauliflower
- Broccoli

Sweeteners

- Coconut sugar
- Date sugar
- Erythritol (sparingly)
- Molasses

US/Metric Conversion Chart

VOLUME CONVERSIONS	
US Volume Measure	**Metric Equivalent**
⅛ teaspoon	0.5 milliliter
¼ teaspoon	1 milliliter
½ teaspoon	2 milliliters
1 teaspoon	5 milliliters
½ tablespoon	7 milliliters
1 tablespoon (3 teaspoons)	15 milliliters
2 tablespoons (1 fluid ounce)	30 milliliters
¼ cup (4 tablespoons)	60 milliliters
⅓ cup	90 milliliters
½ cup (4 fluid ounces)	125 milliliters
⅔ cup	160 milliliters
¾ cup (6 fluid ounces)	180 milliliters
1 cup (16 tablespoons)	250 milliliters
1 pint (2 cups)	500 milliliters
1 quart (4 cups)	1 liter (about)
WEIGHT CONVERSIONS	
US Weight Measure	**Metric Equivalent**
½ ounce	15 grams
1 ounce	30 grams
2 ounces	60 grams
3 ounces	85 grams
¼ pound (4 ounces)	115 grams
½ pound (8 ounces)	225 grams
¾ pound (12 ounces)	340 grams
1 pound (16 ounces)	454 grams

OVEN TEMPERATURE CONVERSIONS

Degrees Fahrenheit	Degrees Celsius
200 degrees F	95 degrees C
250 degrees F	120 degrees C
275 degrees F	135 degrees C
300 degrees F	150 degrees C
325 degrees F	160 degrees C
350 degrees F	180 degrees C
375 degrees F	190 degrees C
400 degrees F	205 degrees C
425 degrees F	220 degrees C
450 degrees F	230 degrees C

BAKING PAN SIZES

American	Metric
8 × 1½ inch round baking pan	20 × 4 cm cake tin
9 × 1½ inch round baking pan	23 × 3.5 cm cake tin
11 × 7 × 1½ inch baking pan	28 × 18 × 4 cm baking tin
13 × 9 × 2 inch baking pan	30 × 20 × 5 cm baking tin
2 quart rectangular baking dish	30 × 20 × 3 cm baking tin
15 × 10 × 2 inch baking pan	30 × 25 × 2 cm baking tin (Swiss roll tin)
9 inch pie plate	22 × 4 or 23 × 4 cm pie plate
7 or 8 inch springform pan	18 or 20 cm springform or loose bottom cake tin
9 × 5 × 3 inch loaf pan	23 × 13 × 7 cm or 2 lb narrow loaf or pâté tin
1½ quart casserole	1.5 liter casserole
2 quart casserole	2 liter casserole

Index

SIMPLIFY AND CUSTOMIZE YOUR DIET!

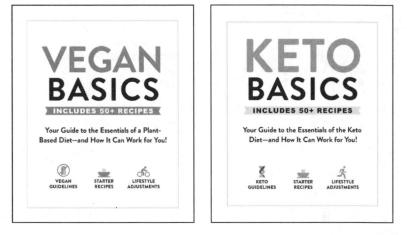

VEGAN BASICS

INCLUDES 50+ RECIPES

Your Guide to the Essentials of a Plant-Based Diet—and How It Can Work for You!

VEGAN GUIDELINES · STARTER RECIPES · LIFESTYLE ADJUSTMENTS

KETO BASICS

INCLUDES 50+ RECIPES

Your Guide to the Essentials of the Keto Diet—and How It Can Work for You!

KETO GUIDELINES · STARTER RECIPES · LIFESTYLE ADJUSTMENTS

PICK UP OR DOWNLOAD YOUR COPIES TODAY!